Pregnancy and Birth: The Conspiracy of Silence

Essential Details they Conveniently Forget to Tell You

BY

CELIA FULLER

Social Media

Connect with me via social media:

https://www.facebook.com/pages/Celia-Fuller-Inspirational-Speaker-Spiritual-Teacher/353354161445344

http://au.linkedin.com/pub/celia-fuller/a1/7b/630

Scan this QR code with your smartphone to visit my websites,

www.wholistic-lifestyles.com.au   www.celia-fuller.com.au

Also by Celia Fuller

The Secret's Out! Men and Sex: Why Women Say No

Kind Words Uplift

Pregnancy and Birth:
The Conspiracy of Silence

Essential details they conveniently forget to tell you.
by Celia Fuller

Published 2014 by CELIA FULLER

All rights reserved. No part of this publication may be reproduced or transmitted in any form or by any means, electronic or mechanical, including photocopying, recording, or by any information storage and retrieval system, without permission in writing from the publisher. All images are free to use or share, even commercially, according to Google and the license purchased from Canstock, Shutterstock and Pixabay at the time of publication, unless otherwise noted. Thank you for respecting the hard work of the author(s) and everyone else involved.

Copyright © 2014 CELIA FULLER
Authors and sources cited throughout retain the copyright to their respective materials.

ISBN: 978-0-9941518-2-7
Photos: Canstock, Shutterstock, Pixabay
Poetry: Celia Fuller
Illustrations: Tasha Wells
Cover Art: Celia Fuller & Tasha Wells

Apologies For Spelling

Spelling is based on American English. If any errors remain then I am happy to hear from you and will rectify any spelling that my editing team did not pick up. Thank you in advance for your care and concern.

Medical Disclaimer

At no point in reading this book should the references to products or alternative health therapists replace the need to first consult a medical practitioner.

The content of this book, *Pregnancy and Birth The Conspiracy of Silence,* including text, graphics, images, and information obtained from contributors and all other content is offered on an informational basis only. No content is intended to be a substitute for professional medical advice, diagnosis or treatment. You should always seek the advice and guidance of a qualified health provider before:

- making any adjustment to any medication or treatment protocol you are currently using
- stopping any medication or treatment protocol you are currently using
- starting any new medication or treatment protocol, whether or not it was discussed in this book.

Information within this book is "generally informational" and not specifically applicable to any individual's medical, emotional or mental problem(s), concerns and/or needs.

If you think you might have a medical emergency, call your doctor or your local health emergency service immediately. If you choose to use any information provided by author Celia Fuller within the pages of *Pregnancy and Birth The Conspiracy of Silence*, you do so solely at your own risk.

This book might contain health and medical-related materials, which some people might find sexually explicit or personally offensive. It is the nature of this book that frank talk about, and discussions on, a variety of topics might occur. The author will attempt to moderate and review content. Purchasing, reading or downloading this book constitutes acceptance of this risk.

Liability

Purchasing or downloading and reading the book *Pregnancy and Birth: The Conspiracy of Silence*, authored by Celia Fuller, is at your own risk.

When using the material in the book, information is transmitted in ways beyond the control of the author. Celia Fuller assumes no liability for the delay, failure, interruption or corruption of any data or other information in connection with use of the digital version.

The content of this book is provided "as is." The author, Celia Fuller, to the fullest extent permitted by law, disclaims all warranties, either express or implied, statutory or otherwise, including but not limited to the implied warranties of merchantability, non-infringement of third parties' rights, and fitness for particular purpose. Specifically, the author, Celia Fuller, makes no representations or warranties about the accuracy, reliability, completeness, or timeliness of the content, software, text, graphics, links, or communications provided on or through the purchasing, downloading, or reading of the book.

In no event shall the author, Celia Fuller, or any third parties mentioned within this book be liable for any damages, including but not limited to incidental and consequential damages, personal injury, wrongful death, lost profits, damages resulting from lost data, business interruption resulting from the purchasing, downloading, or reading based on warranty, contract, tort or any other legal theory, and whether or not the author is advised of the possibility of such damages.

Indemnity

You agree to indemnify, defend, and hold harmless us, our officers, directors, employees, contractors, agents, providers, merchants, sponsors, licensors and affiliates from and against all claims, actions, demands, judgments, losses, and liabilities (including, without limitation, costs, expenses and attorneys' fees) by you or any third-party resulting or arising, directly or indirectly, out of content you submit, post to or transmit through the author's publisher, your use of this book, your connection to this book, your violation of these Terms of Use, or your violation of any rights of another person.

Acknowledgements

A special thank you, to you, my husband, for your kind and considerate understanding as I processed my own issues throughout our pregnancies and children's birth. You remained patient and always did your best to understand me. What a roller coaster ride it has been. Thank you for standing by my side. I cannot finish without thanking and acknowledging you for all your hours of first draft editing and supporting me through the writing process.

To my clients who honored and trusted me with their highly personal stories, I hope I do you justice by writing this book, so that it helps many more women and men through the labyrinth of pregnancy and birth. Thank you for encouraging me to finally write.

Great appreciation goes to Tasha, for helping me with typing and sketches; and Brett, who has been on my case for years to stop talking and start writing. Thanks also to Lyn, who for twenty years has guided me with any IT support and graphics and believed in any project I have started on; and grateful thanks to Michelle for her tireless editing as she constantly worked in the background to make this happen. To Margaret, who for so many years has been a guiding force in my life. To the rest of my friends (you know who you are) who listened to my dreams and also encouraged me to write, I thank you from my heart. Finally last but not least to Mum: your advice, straightforward talking and insight throughout the years have also been embedded within these pages. Thank you.

Dedication

I personally dedicate this book to my boys,
Alex and Ryan.

This has been written to help you understand the women in your world and encourage you both to become loving, patient husbands as you and your future wives or partners go through the life-changing experiences of pregnancy and birth. It is written from a woman's perspective with some inspirational insight gained from your father and other male clients over the years. It is my hope that these words will give reassurance to you both in the years ahead.

Blessed be, Mum.

Contents

Social Media ... ii
Also by Celia Fuller ... iii
Acknowledgements ... viii
Dedication ... ix

Foreword ... 1
Introduction ... 3
Baby Sweet ... 5
Motherhood Trance ... 6

{ 1 } A Body Out Of Control ... 9
    The Test is Positive! ... 10
    What Now? ... 10
    Loss of Libido ... 12
    Give up Planning on Being Superwoman ... 17
    All Consuming Lethargy ... 18
    Loss of Memory ... 19
    Enhanced Smelling Sensations ... 21
    Life Turned Upside Down ... 22
    Urgent Urination ... 24
    Early Breast and Nipple Changes ... 26
    Nausea ... 27
    Crying and Mood Swings ... 30
    Kicking Sensations & Abdominal Discomfort ... 32
    Dreams/ Nightmares – Horror or Truth ... 35
    Baby Belly Becomes Public Property ... 36
    Everyone Has an Opinion ... 38
    My Vagina has Gone Viral! Everyone Wants to See it! ... 40
    No Maternal Instinct ... 41

Bulging Hemorrhoids	43
Whip like Stretch Marks.	45
I am So Over Myself, and this Bowling Ball Walk	46
Ultrasounds	48
OMG! I am so Fat, and It's Not the Baby!	50
Frantic Cooking or Cleaning	51
{ 2 } Physical and Mental Preparation	53
Natural Therapy Preparation Before Birth	54
Wise Hospital Bag	57
Meditation	61
Hypno-Birthing	64
Braxton Hicks Contractions	65
Pre-Labor Visualizations and Exercises	67
Pain Tolerance	71
Support, what does that mean?	73
Oxytocin, the Love Chemical	77
Happy Birth Orgasms	78
Breech Position? Don't Panic, It Can be Changed	78
{ 3 } No Turning Back	83
Mentally Unprepared Men	84
'The Bloody Show' – Mucous Plug (Operculum)	85
Breaking Water	85
Labor Begins	87
The First Stage	87
Established Labor and Birthing –	89
Second Stage Transition	89
What does transition feel like?	90
Get the baby out! Pushing	91
Crowning	92
After Birth Breast Feeding and Bonding	94

Shaky Recovery	98
Needles and Medical Check up	99
Birth of the Placenta – Stage Three Labor	101

{ 4 } Physical Recovery — 103

When Does Bleeding Stop and Sex Start?	104
Medical Checks – Retracting Uterus and Bowel Movements	105
Tearing, Repair – Itchy Stitches	106
Floppy Baby Belly	106
Breastfeeding Clumsiness	107
Engorgement – The Milk Comes	111
Bottle Feeding	115
Cracked Nipples	119
Day Three: Emotional Uproar	120
Lack of Uterus Strength – Pelvic Floor Muscles	121
Prolapse of the Uterus	122
Incontinence	123
Washing and Dressing the Baby	124
Umbilical Cord Care	125
Newborn Black Tar Poo – Meconium	127

{ 5 } A New Family Member — 129

You are Now a Parent	130
Give my Baby Back! Instinctual Protectiveness	131
Mothers and Mothers-in-law	133
Anxiety and Resentment Begin	133
Listening to Advice or Words of Encouragement	135
Fear of Judgment	135
Public Breastfeeding	136
Mother's Groups	137
Breastfeeding Groups	138

Super Mom and Meltdown Moments 139
Sleep When Baby Sleeps 140
Problem Foods and a Developing Digestive System 142
Nervous System Maturing 143
Home Alone with Your Baby 145
Yikes! Now what do we do? 145
My Life is Turned Upside Down 146
Traumatic Births with Medical Intervention 149
Depression Associated with Caesarians 151
Past Sexual Abuse Can Trigger Depression After the Birth 153
Conclusion on Women 155

{ 6 } Don't Forget Your Man 157
A Man's Perspective 158
Birth – Too Many Support People 158
Birth Anxiety 160
Baby Arrival *161*
Home Arrival 162
Crying Begins and the Man Withdraws 163
The Reality Sets In 164
The Fantasy is Crushed 165
Sometimes Your Man Turns into Baby Number Two 166
Put Him to Work 167

{ 7 } Support With Alternative Therapies 169
Bowen Therapy & Acupuncture 170
Massage / Baby Massage 170
Chiropractic / Osteopathic Treatments 171
Wholistic Lifestyle Counseling and Blueprint Healing 172
With Celia Fuller 172
Naturopaths, Herbalists, Homeopaths 173

Bush Flower Essences and Australian Bush Flower Essences	174
In Conclusion	177
About the Author	178
References	179
Also By CELIA FULLER	180
Connect with Me	180
Your Thoughts	180
WEBSITES	180
In Summary	181
A Final Thank You…	181

Foreword

Celia Fuller enjoyed many stages of her pregnancies and the birth of her children, yet was shocked and distressed by other experiences. She realized there were so many areas that women did not openly speak about and this caused her to feel there was a "conspiracy of silence" amongst women in general. Thousands of her female clients backed up this feeling, resulting in Celia's determination to create an open, honest and frank conversation, dispelling many myths and speaking on subjects that otherwise seemed taboo. Empowerment, excitement, confidence and well-being have been the outcome.

Celia has been an Australian wholistic lifestyle consultant, inspirational speaker, natural therapist, counselor, and meditation teacher for over 20 years. Listening to her clients became the backbone of her research. Celia has enjoyed the privilege and honor of listening and treating many young women in various stages of pregnancy and early parenthood. Through their stories, she realized these women struggled to feel reassured or properly prepared for their bodily changes from pregnancy or birth, and especially after birth care, even though they attended prenatal classes. Emotional, mental and sexual challenges caught them by surprise, often creating a sense of isolation, low self-esteem, frustration, and depression. Feelings of failure and not matching up to society's expectations would follow them into the workplace after maternity leave. Doubts about parenting and partnering would consume their mind, resulting in low performance, lack of focus, and reduced inspiration for life, both at work and home. Fulfilling their dreams and passions seemed impossible.

For this reason, this book had to be written.

This book was a pet project that Celia began writing ten years ago. The first draft had been hidden in drawers waiting for her busy life and work schedule to adjust so time could be allocated to complete.

This is Celia Fuller's Gift to the World

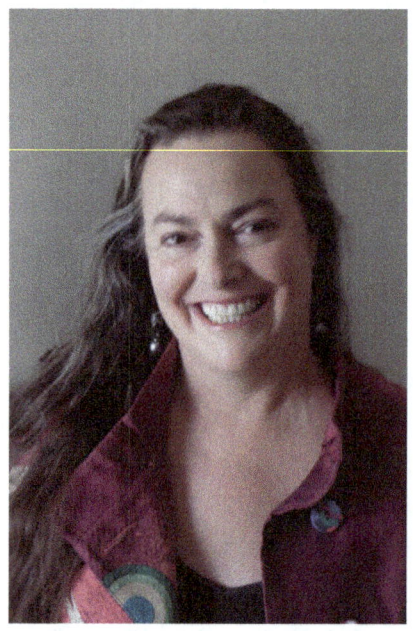

Introduction

This book was written to honor the thousands of women who have walked through my natural therapy clinic door for over twenty years. These women have been open and honest with me about the effects of pregnancy and birth along with the confusion they feel in regards to the whole birthing process and unexpected after care. They speak about the distress they feel in losing a sense of their former self and the sheer difficulty they have in adjusting emotionally. It is my attempt to break the "conspiracy of silence" that seems rampant within the female community and to speak up about those issues that have been hushed.

I wish to minimize the sense of fear, ineptitude, hopelessness, emotional distress, loss of identity, and sheer exhaustion by reassuring others that this is a normal growth process that can be experienced with a sense of empowerment. Knowledge, I believe is the first step to this empowerment.

New mothers come into my clinic with an endless sea of questions that do not seem to have been considered when going to prenatal classes or to doctor visits. The confusion or lack of information seems to range from weird bodily changes, loss of personal space, responsibility, breast feeding difficulties, pressure from mothers groups, difficulties in sexual interest or activity, and even a sense of powerlessness. In my work, I honor and inform those new mothers about alternative choices they can make in relation to natural health remedies, therapies, or psychological support that could support them through this time.

For some women who read this book it may seem as though I have focused upon the purely negative aspects of pregnancy. I do not apologize for this. In light of most women's experiences and emotional perspectives revealed to me, I have realized there is nothing to be gained by covering up or avoiding comments about obvious emotional and mental difficulties through this period. By writing this book I hope to normalize the experience and help each reader feel that they are not alone in their confused feelings about having a baby and their changing relationships.

For those women who seem blessed by boundless joy and contentment with pregnancy and the birth of their child, this book will aid you to empathize with the many women who feel otherwise. Greater understanding and shared experiences amongst the sisterhood will encourage leaps in emotional health and wellbeing for all involved. Each supports the life of the other.

Ladies, share your wisdom. Share it with honesty and truth.

Feelings should not be buried but explored in a caring and insightful way.

Many blessings, Celia Fuller

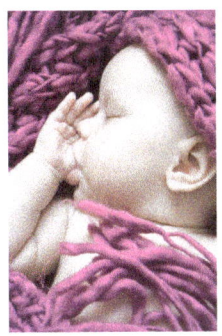

Baby Sweet

A baby's smile lifts the heart,
Releasing moods of the dark.
Gentle innocence swells a mother's breast,
A sleeping child brings out the best.
A mother moves mountains for her child,
Nature it is, a call of the wild.
A new soul born to the physical world,
Proof of oneness has been born.
Man and woman have come together
Joined no matter the forecasted weather.
For good or bad a child is yours
To love, protect from night to morn.
They bring a love, you never knew
Right down deep, in the soul of you.
The blessed gift of a life new born,
Will challenge you forever more.
This gift is yours, so you might grow
Evolving, changing, towards the unknown.
Take heart on this journey, so huge ahead
The demands of heaven, needs to be met.
MAY THE FORCE BE WITH YOU

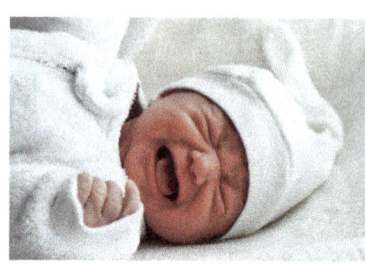

Motherhood Trance

Beware of the motherhood trance,
You wake, you sleep, but never dance.
Time consumed by suckling child,
Screams all night and drives you wild.
Nipples rage with bruised, cracked skin,
Dinner burns, you cannot win.
Elbows deep in runny poo,
I see no bliss but wildlife zoo.
Sleepy state, you see the world,
Washing, cleaning, sleep trance twirl.
Partner wants his bit of flesh
"Rack off mate, hit the deck."
Labor pains are bliss,
Compared to all the shitty mess.
Insane you become beyond compare,
Ranting worse than any nightmare.

Coffee, cake and daytime outings,
All but gone, there is no doubting.
Friends move on but others come,
Mostly other freaked out mums.

Strength drawn from commiseration,
Mums know the truth of your situation.
The going's tough, it never stops,
Pressure builds, your head will pop.
Joy is found, dig down deep,
A child's smile is pretty neat.
When it frowns run a mile,
About to bellow is the child!

{ 1 }

A Body Out Of Control

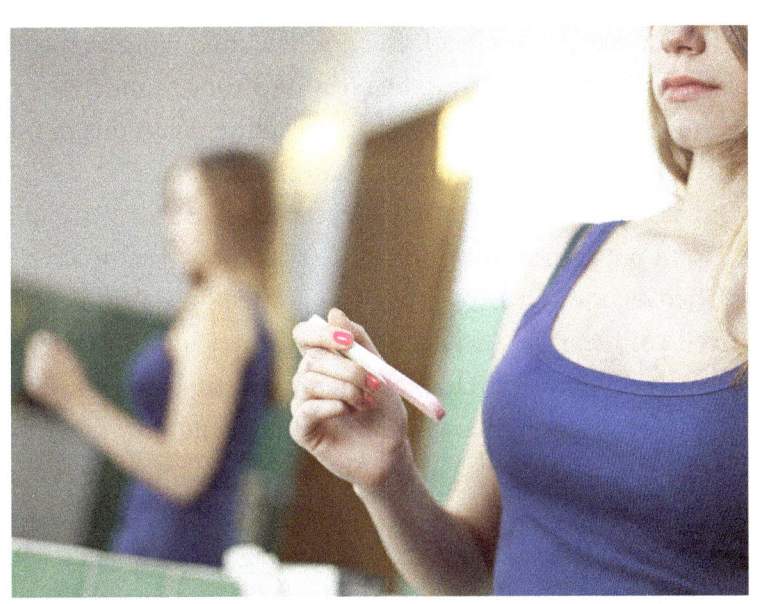

The Test is Positive! What Now?

News of impending motherhood brings with it a flood of emotions. Joy, grief, anticipation, fear, nervousness, excitement, and wonder may consume those early moments. Then reality sets in. What now? What am I up against? What do I have to do? How do I prepare myself?

It always surprises me, when mothers tell women who have not yet conceived all the funny, cute stories of their children's antics. They talk lightly about their pregnancies and leave the yet-to-be mother naïve to what lies ahead. A young woman might be left with stars in her head, convinced a child will enhance her relationship with her partner by creating strong foundations and ensuring a new level of emotional connection. With this in mind she can't wait to begin buying baby clothes.

One day you miss a menstrual cycle, make a secret trip to the shop for a pregnancy test, and before you know what to do next, you discover the test is positive. Congratulations! You have just received your learner's ticket and gained entry into the outer rim of the sacred women's circle. Now that you're pregnant, you attract women who tell stories of morning sickness and how much they struggled. In their voices you still hear an excitement for you, as you have now joined them on a familiar journey. Subjects are kept light and surface-level until you reach a stage of pregnancy where there is no turning back. Then the stories take on a new level of detail. Horror stories tumble out of their mouths—it seems like they take great delight in telling you all the terrifying stories, leaving nicer ones out on purpose.

Through this in-depth sharing you enter a sacred inner circle of a worldwide mother's club, no longer able to turn back to your former life. Your whole world morphs daily. All you see are women with crazy styled prams, lovely devoted fathers, screaming children, and pregnant bellies wearing the latest fashions proudly waddling down the road. It would seem as though the whole universe has conspired to grab you from the clutches of an unfettered life, casting you into a whole new arena. In fact it has! Your world view will never be the same again.

Overnight you become an expert in all things pregnancy, soaking up every available piece of information. You find yourself judging parenting skills of mothers who look irate, stressed, and impatient with their adorable children in tow. You promise yourself you will never be like one of *those* women. Well, as it turns out, those women see the judgmental flicker cross your face and know what's on your mind—they once thought it too. They know it won't be long before you begin to understand what is going on in their lives. You have begun the greatest and most powerful cycle a woman can go through. You have become a partner to creation itself. Life is morphing and unfolding within. But this miracle might not always feel so wondrous. Your body is changing and so is your mind.

As you progress with your pregnancy and the stories come in thick and fast, there may be many shared stories about health and parenting but one area that many women keep to themselves is the subject of sexuality. The emotional and mental anguish a woman can feel as a result of her pregnancy can have an effect on her relationship with her partner, and this can be hard to admit to or discuss openly with others.

For this reason I have begun this book to directly address the problem, as it is not something openly talked about or acknowledged. The subject of sexuality seems to live forever in the darkness and secrecy of relationships, yet has huge and lasting impacts upon how a relationship evolves. It can cause early communication breakdown of an otherwise well suited partnering, resulting in anxiety and stress. This in turn affects our hopes and dreams of the perfect unit welcoming a baby into the mix, hoping it will bring a sense of completion and oneness to the union.

I focus quite a lot on sexuality through pregnancy and beyond, as this is the most commonly raised subject in my consultations. It seems to consume the minds of both the male and female clients. I believe it is probably the most important area of a human's life that needs to feel right, safe, and loving. In my experience, most relationship breakdowns always start from misunderstandings in the bedroom and the subsequent lack of communication that follows.

Loss of Libido

"Why do I try to avoid sex now that I am pregnant?"

Through the process of impregnation a woman's hormones change and adapt to a new life growing within. For some women, having a baby can play havoc on their sex drive. The animal instinct for continuing the species has been met and impregnation practices are no longer required. Considering we are also mammals, our bio-rhythms are not so different to the animal kingdom. Female animals can become quite feral at a male if he shows undue interest in their anatomy. Humans often reflect those same qualities. So there is no need for undue alarm as it is quite natural for pregnant females to lose the urge for sexual activity.

For the male of the species at a primitive level, they are geared to impregnate every female in a group that show signs of ovulation and will mate to ensure the continuing the survival of the species. That explains why males of the human species are frequently in a state of readiness. Nature drives their internal fire. It's also nature in progress when the female begins to internalize all her sexual energy and puts her whole effort into incubating a baby. Alas for men, humans in this day and age are not herd people and society finds it inappropriate for men to attempt to impregnate other women after his wife/girlfriend stops being interested in sex during pregnancy.

If you are faced with a lowered libido and have an amorous husband, do you let him out in the world in an ever-ready state of friskiness? Or, do you act quickly, grab his male appendage by the hand and release his internal fires so he can have power over his thoughts again? I mention this as a gentle precaution as there will be times when pregnancy causes mind-numbing lethargy, obliterating the urge to entertain the slightest bit of sexual activity.

Don't be hard on yourself or question your love. Your hormones are changing and you won't be able to control them. A woman going through pregnancy and after the birth is going to need a whole new approach to foreplay, gentleness, and consideration. The excitement levels will take longer to reach and as a couple you will both need to explore new options together as the days of lust and wild passion have been replaced by a need for a deeper communion of loving. The man will need to work harder to give pleasure and the woman will need to take charge of her sexuality and possibly take the lead to ensure her own comfort. Sadly those wild erotic erogenous buttons that used to work no longer do.

Okay, well no one wants to talk about their glorious sex drive drying up. Literally this is what happens. The body fluids just don't secrete the same. The female pleasure sensations become raw and less sensitive. Men are not always aware that the lack of vaginal secretion usually means a lack of stimulated interest. Since they do not have a vagina, they don't realize vaginal moisture is not just for a man's pleasure and ease of penetration. They might be surprised to learn of the stimulating nature of female secretions and their role in heightening her pleasure.

Dryness might not be so pleasurable for a man but they can still reach orgasm. Women on the other hand can find the dry experience quite irritating, then painful, and even assaulting. The legs clam up, internal anger flares, and women can be emotionally hurt by their partner's continual plunging when they should know it is no longer fun for the woman anymore. Unfortunately the man is not a mind reader and doesn't know this unless the woman TELLS him. If she doesn't tell him he will assume her body sensations are like his own (that she can get off on just about anything). Pregnancy changes everything. It is far better to end the painful intercourse, explain your inability and then find an imaginative way to pleasure the man. Contrary to some women's beliefs, men can get off on the simple hand job and will love his partner even more for understanding his needs.

I know for some of you, the male in your life may be very demanding and may expect you to allow full penetration rather than a hand-job, regardless of your objections, resulting in assault. This is a very difficult subject and one that shall not be explored in this book; however, it is important to acknowledge this scenario does happen to some women, creating even more distress. Personal counseling is highly suggested and self care is of the utmost importance.

Lucky the man whose partner becomes a sexual animal while pregnant

Some rare women can discover a wilder side, as pregnancy for them can increase libido and interest in sex can hit the roof. Partners should be told how lucky they are and to revel in the opportunity for as long as it lasts, as after the birth this experience can wane. Both of you will be the envy of millions who have not experienced this wondrous phenomenon.

I wish I had. A good friend of mine was like that. This lass was a very quiet, God-fearing girl. She told me one day how at a visit to the dentist she felt like leaping from the chair, holding the dentist down, and humping his daylights out. At that stage I had not experienced pregnancy myself and my eyes nearly popped out. She said she felt so wild she could nearly taste it. Those thoughts and feelings consumed her no matter where she went. (When you ask some men they will tell you that's how they feel most of the time.)

Well, I can tell you I was envious of her when I did finally become pregnant. Sadly her story was an unusual one. Within my natural therapy clinic I have mostly heard the sad and grief-stricken perspective regarding a lack of libido. Women would express fear that perhaps they had chosen the wrong partner because their passion has dried up. They were terrified they had made a mistake in choosing their partner, but now they were pregnant it was too late. In my first pregnancy, I too had visited some of those confusing feelings. The guilt alone can really tear you up inside. Thoughts of that kind don't make it easy to share with other people. Internal fears prevent you speaking up to your partner in case they become hurt and defensive. Most women usually have one good friend to talk to, but even then, with thoughts as personal as these, no one is trusted in case these comments find their way back to the partner. Women learn to keep it to themselves. Depression and quiet anguish sets in and the female conspiracy of silence is self-perpetuated.

For these situations, counselling services are beneficial. They are structured so an individual may express all their feelings openly and not fear that confidentiality will be breached. Women don't have to feel alone. Early in pregnancy I sought support about lagging libido, hoping to find a way to activate my interest. When I asked the therapist about this topic I noted her discomfort.

After openly revealing my own internal struggle, she finally let me into her world of experiences on this matter, speaking as a woman and not a practitioner. Through this honest interaction, I discovered that I was not alone. After baby two and the ensuing years of parenting, I decided that I would not perpetuate the silence amongst women by not pretending or not putting on the bright cheery face about the bliss of parenthood. I would share my experiences with brutal honesty, as that is what has helped me thus far. It's not all doom and gloom but this book might make you feel like it is at times, because it's focusing on the topics that have been swept under the carpet.

Intimacy issues around libido and lack of interest can also arise in long-term relationships regardless of pregnancy. For this reason I have written a straight talking relationship rescue guidebook called: *The Secret's Out! Men and Sex: Why Women Say No.*

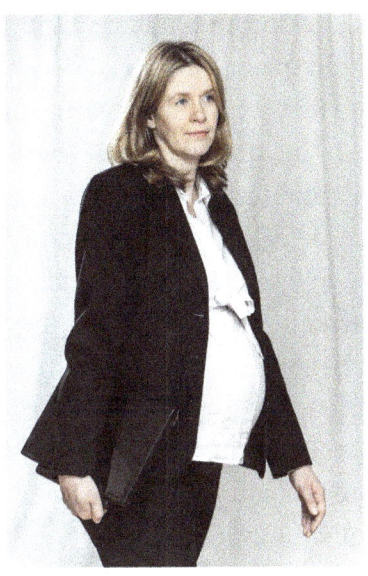

Give up Planning on Being Superwoman

*"I do not know what is wrong with me.
I have lost my mojo."*

You may have great visions of achieving a work/ home balance throughout your pregnancy in an amazing way, unchallenged by the whole experience. If the all-consuming tiredness does not take you out then, the "baby brain" of lost memory or sudden crying events will soon unhinge the best laid out plans. This book gives you permission to accept the process of pregnancy and all the life changes and perspectives that will follow. If you hold on too tight to the dreams of remaining the perfect worker, you might have to face some major disappointments and possibly resent the whole process. This is especially true for women who think they can manage a business, effectively perform in an important corporate role, or plan financially for their maternity leave, expecting this will all happen effortlessly. Pregnancy has a way of disrupting the best held plans.

You might be successful in maintaining a schedule; however, you might have some major emotional breakdowns behind the scenes as you realize how hard you are struggling, just to prove to yourself or others you can do it all. I know, because I went through these same thoughts and feelings too, but exhaustion took its toll and I had to admit defeat. I remember crying with frustration at my failure, yet totally understanding what was happening and finally learnt to surrender to the process. Abandoning building my business allowed me more time to enjoy the different commitments pregnancy brought.

I swam, meditated, walked, and did a huge amount of sleeping. This gave me time to evaluate my life and mentally prepare myself for welcoming a child into the world.

All Consuming Lethargy

"When does the tiredness end? My brain does not work properly and my body is tired all the time. My husband does not know what to do with me. I just want to sleep and sleep and sleep."

This is a familiar experience for many women. The fatigue you can experience, especially with the first child, is mind numbing. Some women might experience this debilitation as early as the first week of pregnancy. Most women will fall under the spell of sleep by the sixth week. This is when new hormones are released within the body, as the egg becomes implanted within the uterus wall. When the egg implants, it finds a vein to attach to and begins to suck out a woman's vital energy. Nutrients and minerals are all siphoned from the mother into the unborn child. A fetus is literally a parasite, a leach! It finds a nice spot, sucks the essence out and then when it's ready, it drops off to be born, only to attach itself to the nipple. Then the whole parasite thing happens again. No wonder new mothers get tired. All their vital energy is going into the child and not a lot is left for their own nourishment. Some women use this as an excuse to overeat while pregnant. It is their way to replenish the stock of lost nutrients.

Eastern mystics from ancient times have often referred to a different more subtle form of energy as being directly responsible for health and vitality of organs, nerves, muscles, brain tissue, and personality. Scientists have now come to understand that all living matter is surrounded by a magnetic field of energy. The mystics have always known this and refer to it as "the life force." This magnetic field surrounds and penetrates our very being, becoming an essential aspect of the human experience. So in response to this, Eastern cultures have developed a variety of exercises designed to increase the life force by drawing energy from the cosmos into the physical body.

The Western world knows these exercises as Yoga, Tai Chi, Qi Gong and Meditation. Any of these exercises can rebuild low pregnancy energy. Martial Arts is under this category as well, but I have only listed the first few as they are slower exercises and usually safe for pregnant women. In other literature you might find the life force energy being referred to as the Prana, Chi or vital energy.

Loss of Memory

"My brain has gone to mush. I can't think straight or remember what I had to remember! When making decisions I can't remember what I am making a decision on."

Memory loss is common and seems to continue even after birth. The hormone changes that occur during pregnancy have a lot to answer for. I have seen highly capable businesswomen come to a screeching halt when they fall pregnant. All their confidence is ripped away due to the brain not being able to work properly. They wonder what has hit them and so do their partners. To women who have chosen to pursue a quieter and simpler way of life and not climb the corporate ladder, rest assured that those who have struggle in exactly the same way as you do. In pregnancy there is no division of social status. All women are placed on an equal footing through the emotional and mental confusion that comes with parenting.

The experience of your brain not working rationally is extraordinary. It can make you feel very incapable and for some women their self-esteem can plunge to a low ebb. Humor is desperately required through this stage and all the others to come. Lift up your head and know that you are not alone. These difficulties can often be enhanced by the use of herbal medicine. Unfortunately for the pregnant women this is not advisable. Some herbs are fantastic but should not be taken while pregnant. Even while breast-feeding some precaution is advised as the herbs will enter the bloodstream and affect the milk. Your practicing complementary health professional will be able to advise you on matters regarding medicinal safety.

With this book I hope to bring to the mass consciousness of women a realization that a path through the jungle can be found. You must learn to be gentle with yourself and dig deep for humor relief. It's helpful if partners are alerted to your possible deficiency. It's a good idea to warn them that the problem might continue on through the toddler years. Your memory will be focused only on the day-to-day safety and nurturing required for your child. Your attention will not usually extend so well to your partner's day at the office, even if you ask him how his day was. Your mind will probably be thinking about bathing time and getting the baby's dinner, rather than fully listening to the response. Women who choose to work or are required to re-enter the workforce early will usually find their faculties returning fairly quickly.

Enhanced Smelling Sensations

"Just the smell of my partner makes me nauseous. I have to catch myself from gagging in front of him!"

"Everything smells disgusting! Cooked food really turns me off."

It is quite common when speaking to women about their sensations of nausea that they connect it to an increased awareness of smell. Day to day smells that were usually ignored or where no real reaction was noted suddenly become the trigger of a wave of intense nausea. The reaction can be a hidden, uncomfortable feeling in the stomach with a slight nasal twitch, to one of horrific proportions of dry retching, gagging, and running for the closest receptacle. This is very difficult when out shopping or passing a restaurant and nostril hairs detect the floating aromas. Before pregnancy these smells would cause salivation but now the mere whiff creates a feeling of faintness with the sensation of an imminent vomit attack.

Even more off putting for a beloved partner is the gag and run from the bedroom trick. While experiencing uncontrollable gagging spells, he lies mystified as to why she left the room with hands covering her mouth. This often occurs simply by waking up and smelling his maleness. Lovemaking fragrances can set it off too. This does nothing for bedroom intimacy or his confidence in his attractiveness and appeal. For some men this can be completely immobilizing and can deter continuing with loving bedroom behavior. This might or might not be welcome news to the pregnant woman in question, but she must be very aware of how her partner feels about this. He will need a lot of reassurance that she does indeed find him attractive at <u>all</u> other times, just not at the moment as she is feeling so sensitive to her environment. A great way to help the man feel loved and not rejected is the good old fashioned hand job in the shower trick. While under running water, smells seem to dissipate and mixed with the soap it could be quite pleasant. Just don't look at the end product or that can bring on a reaction too. Alternatives to soaps and perfume smells can include massage oils.

Most men will welcome any consideration of his needs in such a way. He will still feel loved and even amazed at how simple his needs can be met. He may even consider that this pregnancy thing could be fun for him as well. For those who hesitate to go to such measures and feel guilty for not providing the full penetration experience for your husband, rest assured that I have made a point to talk to many men on this subject. Their common response is, "They are simply happy that their needs are being met in other ways."

I want to stress at this point that if you at any time feel that this behavior threatens your personal space and you just cannot bring yourself to do these things for your man, then do not proceed. This is the time for respectful communication. These ideas are only put forth as a way to move through any guilt or sense of failure that can arise when pregnant. They are also to help partners who can be so deeply affected, often negatively at this precious time.

Life Turned Upside Down

"I am so scared by the changes in me."

Women often expect that the man in their life will be considerate and patient. But they are not in our bodies and have absolutely no clue whatsoever of how the body can betray our perceptions of ourselves, our sexuality and our relationships. With pregnancy everything changes in wild ways. Nothing is the same anymore. There is hope that once the baby is born it will get better. But it won't ever be the same as the past. All your experiences are changing and evolving.

The human mind often fears change and will fight against it in order to cling to the old version of one's self. We live in the past and cling to the hope that the future will be re-enacted as the past once was. Pregnancy is no different and can cause the fight/flight reflexes to become over-stimulated, creating great anxiety. Bringing a child into the world requires personal adaptation.

Acceptance of mammoth proportions is required for this new phase in your life. This recognition needs to come from not only the mother but the father too. Many women are already aware that change is required. Fortunately for the survival of the human species we have no real idea just how much everything changes until we are right in the middle of it. We must learn to be calm and gentle on ourselves and take it one day at a time. Men struggle desperately to understand the required changes ahead. What he does not understand, he sweeps under the carpet and leaves it there. He does not look at it again. He does not speak to his mates about his wife's gagging behavior and the lack of interest she has. At the bar they might make some light jokes but they do not deal with it in a deeper fashion. Anything that seems to have a highly emotional quality to it makes a man shrink. He mulls over it quietly and intensely in the shed or when he can find a quiet moment to reflect. Do not fall into the trap and assume he is not trying to decipher these mystifying changes in you. He will be thinking about it flat out. Anything that threatens the bedroom antics will be thought about! If he does not come up with an answer of how to fix it, you will never know his deeper thoughts and feelings on the matter. Just remember a man is not a mind reader and will need you to attempt to fill him on the details and let him know how you are feeling.

Having spoken in general terms I must say that the male stereo type is changing and men are more proactive in seeking out information and their feelings are spoken of more freely. There are also women who refuse to reveal the true depth of how they are feeling or coping. They fear they are a failure as they compare themselves to all the other women running around looking like super women, but struggling underneath that façade.

Urgent Urination

"I panic if I have to go somewhere new, as I don't know where the closest toilet is."

"Is it normal to spend all night in the loo?"

Some ladies will be more affected than others. It is common knowledge that the urge to urinate increases quite early in pregnancy. A standard question from my doctor was, "Have you been trotting off to the toilet a lot lately?"

"Trotting off to the toilet?" I'd screech in reply. "I spend half my bloody life there! Some nights as soon as I have returned to bed I have to turn around and do it all again! One night it was so extreme, I resorted to sitting on the toilet, pillow wedged between my shoulder and my head trying to get some sleep in between each session. How ridiculous is that! By day I would walk around like a zombie just trying to get over it", I answered in a frustrated, near hysterical reply. Night after night this can be your story. No one warned me it could become so life consuming.

A weak bladder in some people might be the cause for a much greater urgency and frequency than others. When the baby grows larger, room to maneuver in the abdomen lessens, creating a higher incidence of low bladder control. Occasional feet or elbows jammed into the bladder will demand a near sprint to the closest toilet. Panty shields are a great way to give you a little more comfort and security for these emergencies. Second babies are worse as the pelvic floor muscles may not be as strong as they once were.

Throughout your pregnancy it is a good idea to do a regular series of pelvic floor exercises.

Pelvic floor exercises

- When urinating, practice stopping the flow for ten seconds and then resume again. You can do this twice in the one flow and then allow nature to take its course. Do this each time you go to the toilet or as often as you can remember. If you can remember!

- While sitting or standing, squeeze your anus as though you are trying to stop a bowel movement. Move forwards, then squeeze the muscles responsible for cutting off the flow of urination. Once squeezing tight, hold this position for seven to ten seconds. As before repeat this as often as you can remember.

These exercises are very important to continue after birth. They strengthen all your muscles associated with the bladder, anus and vagina. They will also tone a deeper set of muscles in the lower abdominal region. If you continue these exercises throughout your life, confidence with your sexual prowess and prevention of early onset of aged incontinence can be the outcome.

Early Breast and Nipple Changes

*"Why have my nipples gone dark?
Will they return to normal?"*

Breasts can enlarge quite a lot during pregnancy as the new hormones are instructing your body to begin preparing for the baby's arrival. They will return to normal size after breastfeeding ceases. Sometimes it might seem like there is less tissue volume than before, suggesting that somehow the baby has sucked all the breast tissue out from behind the skin. Breasts may appear to hang lower and have some wrinkles as the breast tissue fat has lessened and this is usually more evident after consecutive births. This does not stop you from being a successful breastfeeder.

It is quite normal to become aware of changes in nipple color and size. The color changes can occur in the early weeks and will continue to darken closer to birth. They may lighten a little after birth, but usually they remain in the darker shade. This is one way to tell that a woman has been pregnant before. The raised glands may become more prominent and your nipples become more erect.

The glands are the little lumps surrounding the nipple and sit within the areola looking like pimples.

Your nipples can become quite sensitive and tender. In preparation for breastfeeding it is suggested that you begin manually squeezing, pinching and pulling on them on a regular basis to toughen up the nipple tissue. Your partner can be encouraged to take part in this nipple physiotherapy as a form of foreplay. That is, of course, if you manage to not slap him due to their sensitivity. Doing this early can prevent nipple splitting and cracking when breastfeeding starts. There is no guarantee cracking won't happen, but it certainly is a good preparation both mentally and physically.

Leaking Nipples – Milk can begin leaking out of the nipples as early as three months; however, it is more common to be advanced in pregnancy before breasts begin to leak. In the early stages and before birth, milk that comes out is usually colostrum. In case you are in the minority that produces milk early, you should be prepared with breastfeeding pads, otherwise you could end up experiencing soggy bedsheets through the night or wet patches appearing on your shirt through the day.

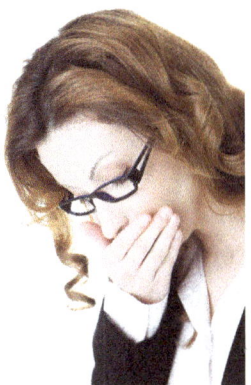

Nausea

"I have to carry a vomit bag with me everywhere I go as some days I could vomit all day. Is there any way I can stop it?"

"I don't get morning sickness; mine comes at night."

A parenting manual would not be complete if we did not address the debilitating reality of morning sickness. Hormonal changes from fetal growth seem to cause an overwhelming sense of nausea. The average time reported for onset of symptoms is around the six-week mark due to the fetus implanting into the uterus wall. Prior to that occurring, the egg has been continuously dividing at a phenomenal and complex rate. When the implantation occurs, the fetus is then attached to your blood supply and energetically connected to your whole system. Common relief from this sensation occurs after the second trimester. Some women become instantly sick within a day of conception, while others vomit every day of their pregnancy. The most fortunate go through nine months unscathed. Often morning sickness can resume at night.

Clients of all ages have generously passed on common remedies that eased their symptoms. I pass them on now to you, hoping you will find something that provides ease.

Ginger tablets are used by quite a lot of people with varying degrees of success. Ginger beer can also be of assistance. Some say Coca-Cola has been their savior. Many women find they gravitate to greasy junk foods to create a lining on the stomach, and swear on its effectiveness.

As you can see, most of these suggestions are high in sugars or fats and not recommended to consume in large quantities. I suggest some discipline here, as it doesn't take much to pack on weight when pregnant, and it might not always come off as easily as we'd like. I know! I ate chips and ginger beer. Not always, but enough to allow cellulite to gain quite a foothold. They did give me blessed relief, but at what cost? I can honestly state, and thousands of women will agree, the low body image you can experience after having your baby can be an overwhelming negative experience that might hang around for years, especially if weight loss eludes even though breastfeeding. Only you can decide if a quick grease or sugar hit is worth the long-term ramifications.

Consuming greasy food might be the only path to ensure a stable stomach and remain a functional member of the family unit. This is even more imperative if you have other kids to look after. It's so easy to become consumed with a sick feeling and really aggravated if those close to you demand that you function as your usual joyful, positive self. Well, you can forget that. It does not happen. An upcoming mother will do anything to just stop these feelings, thinking, "Stuff the weight! I'll deal with that later."

Avoiding weight gain from unwise food choices is possible. There are travel sickness bands that can be placed over specific points on the wrist that act like acupuncture. They also have the same effect on morning sickness, with many women proclaiming effectiveness through the entire gestation period. Personal trials found the band alleviated the intense symptoms, with only some discomfort remaining. Greasy food filled the void.

I noticed my worst days of nausea were always associated with a lack of recent bowel motion. Constipation had a huge part to play with my increased nausea. As soon as my bowel motions resumed, the nausea either instantly stopped or diminished considerably. This made sense to me due to training in iridology as part of my naturopathic studies. Iridology is a technique based on the iris of the eye being considered a general map of the body and its health and works on the premise that bowel function is the central organ behind all our physical dysfunctions. By looking at the iris eye map, a practitioner sees that all the nerves and body organs are attached to the bowel regions. Blockages in the bowel cause toxic fumes to escape into the system resulting in nausea. For some readers, this may not sound logical but if you were to visit a naturopath, they would be able to show you a chart that will demonstrate what I have just said. To me the truth is in the results. By this understanding alone I was able to diminish my own nausea symptoms and then later on for my clients. I suggest you give more attention to the area of constipation to help with nausea relief. Perhaps you too can find extra relief in this method.

Tiredness can become another factor for an onset of dreadful nausea. This usually happens in the early evening when the day is finished and you are too tired to arrange the evening meal. The body becomes dreadfully fatigued after a long day. It seems fatigue causes a queasy sensation to arise. Even though hunger pervades the senses, your body sends signals that it will reject the food if you eat. Nausea becomes all-consuming and sleep evades as the stomach feels like it is eating itself away. Many women usually express a need to only eat the food they crave. No other food will suppress the uncomfortable feeling. This is the state of mind a woman gets into before she eats greasy food, just to put some kind of lining on the stomach. When eaten, it is a blessed relief, allowing her to enjoy the rest of the evening.

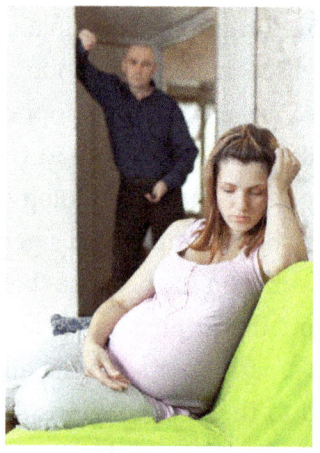

Crying and Mood Swings

*"I'm crying over silly things all the time.
Why do I feel so depressed?"*

"I am so angry. My husband is ducking his head and avoiding me, but I just can't seem to stop my tongue from lashing out at him."

Radical emotional shifts and changes coming to the fore during pregnancy are usually well addressed in the multitude of books on the market. It is common knowledge that women move through many emotional states due to hormonal changes. It is also a time where a huge mental and emotional adjustment is demanded.

Nature demands that a woman must grow up quickly as she only has nine months to make this sudden change. She must mature and be totally responsible for the care and nurturing of a new being on this planet. Even though a woman may have a partner, it is not usually expected that he must adjust nearly so much as the woman. Sure, they have to see life from a new perspective but they usually stand back, seeking the woman's help and guidance. How can a woman give that guidance when she flounders around with mothering, birth, changes in sexuality and still cooking, cleaning, feeding, waking up at all times in the night and then moving through each day in a numb, coma-like state.

Women, I believe, intuitively know that to have a child means huge sacrifices to their freedom. This inner knowing sets off all kinds of reactions in the female psyche. They know intrinsically that to have a child means the loss of her former identity and a metamorphosis into a new person. This is scary and threatening, making it natural for her to feel out of sorts, easy to anger or show impatience. The body is changing and as the baby grows her movements feel heavy and cumbersome, and each day she tries to cover up groans and grimaces. Some days the baby kicks so hard she feels bruised from the inside out.

Don't be surprised if your reactions are a little on the wild side. Partners will have to move out of close proximity. The paradox is, if they attempt to withdraw, they will be punished with snarls and growls for not supporting your emotional neediness at this time. They cannot win in this scenario.

For ***male readers,*** it is important now that you show gentler, emotional support. A hug does not mean you instantly have to drag the woman to the bedroom. When she snaps at you, it is not appropriate for you to leave the home, tail between the legs, and go moping to the public bar. You'll only suffer worse when you get home.

You need to be available to listen to her thoughts and feelings if she wants to talk. If your partner is talking all about the birth, covering subjects already gone over ten times before, then do it again. This is your partner's way of processing all the changes ahead and within her body. She needs to talk about it to try to find a resting place within her psyche and make peace with the process.

Crying over ridiculous things is very unnerving for both partners. The whole process unhinges, as her mind no longer feels like her own. She is out of control. Do not be surprised if she literally cries over spilt milk, a spoon dropping to the floor, placing objects in the fridge when they belong in the cupboard or turning up late to a coffee date.

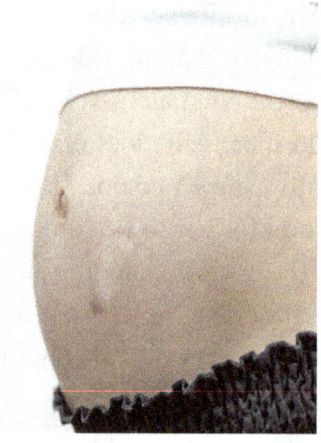

Kicking Sensations & Abdominal Discomfort

"I can't sleep at night. I feel so uncomfortable with reflux. Why do I have pain down my leg?"

Anticipation increases waiting for that first kick or baby movement. An eternity seems to pass before you are rewarded with the pleasure of the first physical proof of life, the child moving within. This experience anchors the pregnancy and changes you. The developing baby no longer exists on a screen, seemingly separate from you. For both you and your partner, it begins a new level of intimacy and bonding followed by intense planning. Detectable baby movements occur around 5-6 months after gestation.

Those first sensations are often described as butterfly wings moving around and tickling the inside abdomen. Those feelings gradually increase until you experience indisputable kicking actions. It's not long after this new development that your sleep becomes constantly disturbed. The baby sleeps during the day mostly remaining motionless, only to perform somersaults throughout the night. Your lack of sleep causes more fatigue, making the day ahead drag on with you in a trance like state.

Their favorite place to kick seems to be the bladder. So expect multiple night-time excursions to the toilet. The most disconcerting place for a foot to kick is when the baby is in birth position, head down bottom up, with the foot plunging directly into the liver and gallbladder, just under the right ribcage or the pancreas underneath the left ribcage. Those major organs have a vital part to play in digestion, yet the baby's foot seems to love pushing on your internal parts with acrobatic maneuvers. At times you can spend days in total discomfort constantly trying to push the foot away to gain some nausea reprieve. When the baby is positioned high up in the abdominal cavity, especially in the last trimester, you can become extremely short of breath with increased reflux and heartburn.

At other times the baby might sit deep in the pelvic cavity in breach position, activating the large sciatic nerve that threads its way down the leg. Sharp bursts of leg and hip pain or deep aching with bursts of throbbing down your legs can go on for weeks. Night after night, and even through the day, pain becomes ever-present, not abating until baby decides to move off the immediate area. Sciatic pain is not always from the baby's position; this can be a result of softening ligaments during pregnancy, a natural process of birth preparation. Massage can be very beneficial to help alleviate some of this discomfort.

The sensation of the baby moving is not always pleasurable for all women; distaste and fear can increase when movements become quite visible. By the time seven to eight months roll along, it's usual to witness the whole abdomen shifting, with the little footprints or elbows protruding from the rounded drum-like shape. It can feel like an alien lives within and is taking over. Rolling, pushing, and pulling keeps you awake at night, causing multiple levels of discomfort with no control over the process. By the end of eight months a reprieve from activity is usual as there is less room within the uterus for ease of movement. The baby by now is slowing down and remaining in the birth position. If the baby lies in the breach position, don't be surprised if it suddenly flips over last minute.

If your baby doesn't move a lot through the pregnancy, don't panic as this may be indicative of its overall temperament. If worry overtakes you, speak with your doctor or midwife, and scans will ease your anxiety and inform of any problems. I believe in women's intuition and gut feelings. If you are really concerned, push for a scan and more investigation and don't allow medical personnel to placate or treat you like an over anxious first mom. It's far better to make sure than find out a problem existed when it's too late. Male doctors and women who have not carried a baby have no idea how a women can feel in relation to her intuitive connection to the baby. So often I hear the stories of women being ignored but in the end they were right, sometimes with a sad outcome.

It's your body and your baby, don't let anyone boss you.

Dreams/ Nightmares – Horror or Truth

"I keep having dreams that something is wrong with my baby."

"I notice in my dreams I am paranoid around the baby, making me scared about how I will parent."

"My baby visited me in a dream last night and spoke with me."

Sometimes reoccurring dreams may alert you to something not being quite right with your body, the pregnancy or with the baby. This can be a truth couched in reality or an overanxious paranoia creating horror scenarios in your dreams. It is important that you don't act with major anxiety, running to the doctor every time you have a dream. It is quite common to experience bad dreams during pregnancy, as the subconscious mind reacts to sensations of fight and flight instincts, thus creating all manner of worrying images. You can have an array of really lovely, powerful, life affirming dreams also.

Many clients, and even I, have experienced the profound and wonderful process of the baby introducing itself in a mental telepathic form. This can be through symbolic dreams or direct dreams where the child reveals its general nature and disposition, later proving to be 100 percent accurate. Extraordinarily, you may even be told in your mind and shown by images, in the awake or dream states, the life path of the child including gifts and inbuilt skills. This in itself is a marvel, creating a deeper bond between mother and child.

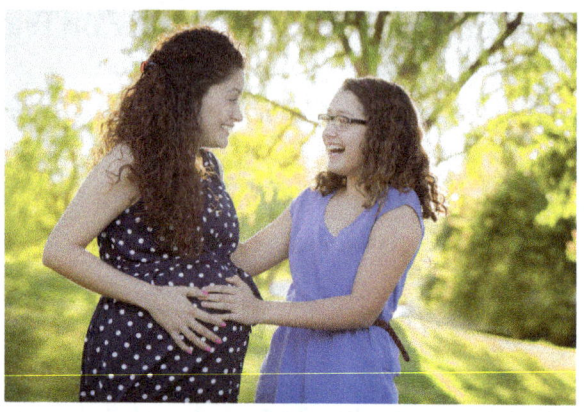

Baby Belly Becomes Public Property

"Why do strangers think they can just walk up and touch my baby belly? I feel like my body has become public property."

"How do I make them stop?"

What is going on in people's minds when they think they can just lunge forward, demanding to touch, pat, or feel your baby belly? Random strangers, both male and female, suddenly morph into psycho stalkers just waiting for a chance to touch your precious cargo. One moment you are an unknown person going about daily business, next minute you have become the center of attention and seemingly public property without the right to say, No! My first response to this problem is to reassure and maintain that it's perfectly okay to say no and tell them to stop. If you feel compelled to slap a hand, then do it. Honor your instincts, and take action if needed; alternatively, reach out and touch their stomach in return. They will retract in horror but it can certainly get the message across. You might have even been one of those offenders in the past, without having realized the weirdness of such behavior.

It is the strangest experience becoming public property when prior to pregnancy only a handful of people were allowed in your intimate zone. Closest family and loved ones might kiss, cuddle, and hold you, but other people— even friends—are not encouraged to enter your personal bubble. How many people, do you know would just walk close to you pre-pregnancy and start grabbing at your stomach or asking to stroke it? Not many. In fact, you would probably think they were very strange and try to avoid them after doing such a thing. You might even think they are entering the space to introduce intimate relations. Possible reactions can explode in wild and unexpected ways, with sudden leaping backwards, arms crossing over the stomach in protection, turning away, or giving an involuntary squeal of horror or shout out in warning. Uncensored reaction might potentially hurt or horrify others because they have not processed their unconscious decision to enter your personal space and touch your belly. Why does this happen? you might ask. Protective responses are completely understandable as your role is to protect the unborn young. Even when not pregnant, a woman might feel quite vulnerable if someone was to grab at her abdomen. In this area of your anatomy, major organs sit unprotected below the ribcage, so we naturally curl over or retract if someone suddenly reaches out. This is the first place you are taught to protect in martial arts. So when your pregnancy is strikingly evident, you have no possible way to curl away in protection or prevention from the baby shape presenting to the world. Your only option becomes defense by attacking. This can cause a lot of family distress and anxiety, especially when the mother-in-law lays claim to the unborn baby.

When you think about it, in a way, the protruding baby bulge and subsequent man-handling is the baby's first introduction to the world and the varied styles of people he/she will eventually encounter. For those who understand about the human magnetic field that science has proven exists, it makes more sense that you would want to shield and protect your child from people and their negative energy exchange. That is why some days you might feel comfortable for the touch and other days not. Honor yourself and your intuitive awareness.

As a society we are fascinated with the look of a pregnant belly and all that comes with it. Young women are awed and scared of what they see and try to become more connected and knowledgeable about what the future holds for them when they are in the same situation. They do this by asking to feel the abdomen. Often their face will be filled with awe and fear combined. Many men find a pregnant lady very sexy and are equally fascinated by the concept of life moving inside. They may be less inclined to approach and touch. It's usually the older women who think they have the right, since they have been through the process themselves. In some weird subconscious way it might be a tribal behavior of welcoming the child to the group. I think an independent study on this could be interesting as it's such a common phenomenon. I wonder how many animal species show the same level of interest in the unborn baby belly.

In summation, it's your body and you choose who touches you!

Everyone Has an Opinion

"I feel like I have lost my own identity."

There is a distinct feeling of losing individual identity once pregnant. Not only are people grabbing and touching your belly but all the conversations seem to morph into wild baby talk, labor stories, wives tales, and a lot of opinions and suggestions. It seems as though people have forgotten you actually have a mind and life of your own and are more than just a baby-making machine. It's as though all the years of hard work invested in developing a career is null and void. All history is wiped clear as though you are now finally doing your life's purpose as a female. This whole scenario can be completely frustrating for women, especially for those who see their work as their identity.

A normally reliable body has betrayed all your well thought out plans, exacerbating the feeling of lost identity. Wanting to sleep when you have to work, exercise routines abandoned by falling asleep on the couch soon after getting home, and dinner parties abandoned as nausea and body discomfort is battled. All these events drive home that your body now has two owners. You are now dictated to from the inside, sucked dry by some foreign alien that you are supposed to feel masses of love towards. Instead, a lack of ease consumes the mind as it ponders on the changes you have so far implemented and the future ones you have to make. Convincing yourself that your identity will be reclaimed once the baby is born becomes your mantra.

It does not finish here; wait, there is more to come!

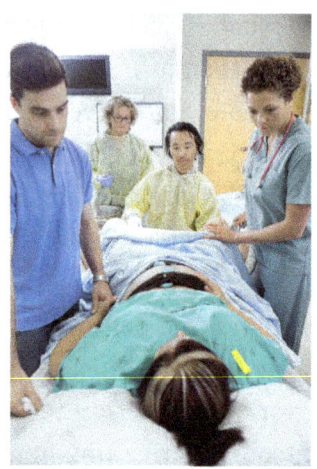

My Vagina has Gone Viral! Everyone Wants to See it!

"I am so embarrassed and mortified that doctors, nurses and midwives all want to peer under my skirt."

Pregnant and welcomed into the halls of fame, your body becomes the subject of a huge scientific experiment. Poking, peering, prodding, scans, ultrasounds, and more poking and prodding seem the order of the day. A vagina that was once a place of mystery and mystique, offering gifted viewing only to the initiated of intimate partners, now has everyone thinking they can have a go. Humiliation usually flushes the face and body as each new person takes a peek, or probes some cold instrument inside, or decides to finger your bottom hole to determine the state of your pregnancy.

All you want to do is look the other way and pretend it is not happening, or to bash the offending hand. It's natural to feel so uncomfortable because you have been trained throughout your life to keep those parts of yourself private from others and not let people touch down there unless you have an early medical condition, or wish to enjoy the art of love and intimacy. Sadly, the closer that birth encroaches, the more vigorous those inspections become. After birth it just gets better and better—not!

I know this sounds scary, but I believe it's better to be prepared, because sometimes a huge feeling of violence can overcome you, especially when trainee hospital staff want to stick their fingers in your abdomen, pummeling your baby, and it bloody hurts. When subjected to the medical system, needing their care can sometimes cause you to feel powerless to pull up a staff member on how they approach your body. However you are well within your rights to speak up and ask for gentler consideration or even say, No. Trainee male doctors or nurses are the worst as they often feel nervous to do this work, so their bedside manner suffers. They become matter of fact, robotic and at times downright rude. In fact, anyone who has themselves have not been pregnant and needs to palpate your abdomen or do vaginal inspections has no idea how uncomfortable and painful the process is or how angry a mother can become due to her protective instinct for the unborn child.

In our Western world we are fortunate to have well trained professional staff on hand to help us through every stage of pregnancy. Part of our success in medical knowledge has been gained from probing, prodding, and peeking in the nether regions. So I suppose we have to keep a balanced view on our reactions and keep the flared tempers in check.

No Maternal Instinct

> *"I don't think I am ready to be a mother because I do not feel excited or maternal. What is wrong with me? I don't want to talk about babies all the time."*

Guilt and concern rage within pregnant women when they compare themselves to other women in the same situation. They listen to all the excited stories of clothes bought, progress reports of the nursery preparation and the ultimate purchase of car seats and prams. Surprisingly, in my clinic, there seems to be a large percentage, even up to 70 percent, of women who feel a distinct lack of excitement or engagement in the process towards motherhood. It made me wonder if the percentage is even higher and women feel a need to fake emotions that are not actually there, contrary to media presentations.

Not only do women complain of a lack of maternal instinct, but they also comment on how impatient they have become by all conversations seeming to morph from intelligent analysis of life and what is going on in the world into constant focus on the pregnancy and children. They feel their individuality has lost importance, relegated to listening to a constant supply of birthing anecdotes. Frustration and depression follow as they feel trapped in a cycle they did not know they had chosen just by becoming pregnant. Losing a sense of self-identity and individuality was not on the agenda.

I belonged to the 70 percent and was disappointed by my lack of maternal frenzy and excitement. In my young single years, I oozed with gushing enthusiasm over baby clothes and toys, and spent many a waking hour dreaming about the joy a child would bring to my life. After the initial thrill of knowing I was pregnant, the expected emotions never surfaced! It was like my body had been taken over by a robot; I was unemotional and unprepared. I was only driven to begin baby shopping after my father-in-law made a phone call months after gifting us some money to see what we actually purchased. He was a little stunned to learn, by the seventh month, I had not even begun. This made me realize that perhaps it was expected of me to begin some form of preparation. My mind then drifted into a state of concern about my future mothering skills.

Years later I reflected on my attitude, when woman after woman seeking counseling or natural therapy treatments expressed to me they shared this same disengaged state. It became apparent this state of mind is more common than publicly stated and women experience guilt and anxiety through pregnancy when they need not. Sharing this realization with new clients helped reduce their anxiety.

If you feel this way, don't beat yourself up about it. Your mothering capacity will not be affected. Lowered exhilaration comes from a body internalizing life energy for baby growth and a lack of enthusiasm will not affect your future mothering capacity or ability to love. If conversations are extremely baby orientated then gently tell your friends that you would like to talk about something else. Introduce a new topic and challenge the women in your life to accept your needs to be seen as more than a baby incubator. Years later this will help them develop the skills and confidence to speak up also.

Bulging Hemorrhoids

"I have a sore anus with lumpy bits."

"What is bulging out of my back passage?"

*"OMG! I have developed balls!
They are purple and hanging from me!"*

Sadly it's a common experience for women to experience unusual lumpy protrusions from the anus when pregnant or years later due to pregnancy. These protrusions are called hemorrhoids and are blood vessels from the rectum that have become quite swollen. Formation is more common in the third trimester due to the baby being positioned heavily in the lower abdomen, placing extreme pressure on pelvic veins sitting above the anus and vagina. Constipation can be another contributing factor.

Hemorrhoids mainly remain hidden within the anus while other times they start to protrude out to the surface. Some clients have spoken of horrifying, mind-numbing stories of their hemorrhoids appearing like testicles hanging freely. Fortunately, and to their great relief, they eventually retracted after giving birth, and it is rare to have such large sacs showing externally. The most irritating aspect of hemorrhoids is the discomfort. Walking and sitting becomes difficult and the internal itch is challenging. Some bleed, adding to your apprehension.

Labor is another time when hemorrhoids might activate. This is due to the extreme downward pressure exerted upon the anus as part of the birth process. If you experience hemorrhoids in pregnancy or birth and they naturally retract, they might reappear with age or when constipated. Once blood vessels are weakened they become susceptible to new events.

Don't panic, you don't have to remain like this forever. If they don't disappear soon after the birth I suggest you seek medical intervention.

To help avoid or reduce hemorrhoids there are a few options.

*Avoid constipation through pregnancy and especially immediately after the birth by eating raw foods and those high in fiber. Drink lots of water to stay hydrated, allowing the fiber to move freely and easily within the bowel and keeping the fecal matter soft.

*Witch hazel cream is fantastic to eliminate irritation and assist the blood vessels to retract. This can be used externally on the outer surface and by way of inserting small amounts within the anal opening.

*Bottom wiping should be with a softened unscented towelette as normal toilet paper is quite rough when you feel so uncomfortable. There are pre-medicated wipes with witch hazel on the market that can ease discomfort. Ice and cold compresses might ease the swelling and help the vein to retract.

*Keep moving; exercise helps all the muscles of the pelvic area remain strong and supple along with increased circulation. Never underestimate the power of the pelvic floor muscle exercises.

Special note: Before using any of these remedies and ideas it is best to seek a medical practitioner.

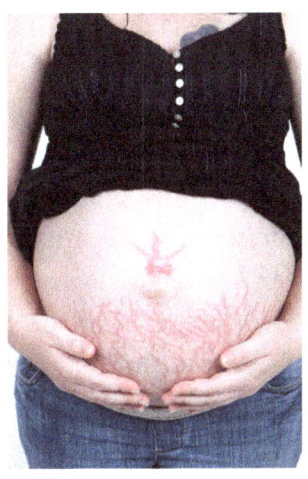

Whip like Stretch Marks.

"My stomach itches like crazy and I have these ugly lines everywhere."

Be prepared, most women will end up with some stretch marks even after using every oil and skin preparation imaginable to prevent them. If nothing else, all that stroking of the stomach is great for your developing child, often ensuring a calmer constitution. So do not let me diminish your enthusiasm in trying to lessen the possibility of stretch marks. Stretch marks at first appear dark reddish purple in color and can look as though you have been whipped. Upon closer inspection you can actually see how the skin has lost its capacity to stretch with thinning skin appearing in lines and striations across the belly and over the hips. Sometimes they can be seen on breasts, the inner thighs, or over the buttocks. Stretch marks when forming can feel itchy.

Pregnant women are not the only ones who get stretch marks. Some males and females have a higher genetic pre-disposition to them. You fit this category if stretch marks have already appeared on your skin from earlier weight gain or through rapid growth phases in adolescence, or if your siblings have them. Don't panic, in time the ugly purple color lightens and eventually they become silvery small lines. The drawback comes when floppy skin remains even after reducing back to your pre-pregnancy weight.

As a natural therapist I have seen many women in a state of undress and have been amazed at how well most of them bounce back and still look great, even with a few lines that tell the story of their pregnancy. So have faith, you can still look beautiful and sexy once repair is completed.

I am So Over Myself, and this Bowling Ball Walk

"I feel like I am crushing my baby's head.
It feels like it's going to fall out!"

"I am so over this bowling ball between my legs."

The new walk you have to adopt when heavily pregnant does not help hemorrhoids. Some women can feel gross and ugly through the heaviest part of pregnancy due to their walk, becoming so unfamiliar, awkward and uncomfortable. Yet other women proudly waddle like a graceful pelican, chest and abdomen strutting out to the world, but even for them there comes a time when they just want it to stop. The pressure of the baby's head causes a new level of incontinence and you can no longer walk in a straight line. You literally have to throw your legs slightly to the side as you walk just to get around the sensation of the head in the way. It's easy at this stage to think you might crush your baby.

I remember reading an article about a woman conveying to her husband how it felt to be heavily pregnant and then go into labor.. Each trimester the man should imagine walking around with a progressively larger and heavier bowling ball stuck up his anus. When it comes to labor, imagine an umbrella being pushed up inside and gradually opened. It did make me smile and I thought to myself it would certainly help the man feel part of the process and perhaps become more mindful of his partner's discomfort and need for emotional support through these trying times, especially closer to the birth date.

By the end of the last trimester women are so sick of being in this condition. Sick and tired of not being able to breathe or get up from or into a chair or bed easily, they want to reclaim their body. The baby keeps organ kicking, they can't walk easily without shooting pains firing off from the pubic bone area. Milk might be leaking from the nipples, staining favorite clothes, and they worry about people staring at them in fear at any moment they will lose their waters. Indigestion and heartburn becomes their new friend, arriving each night just before bed, causing more sleep deprivation. They feel hot, flushed and flustered, never thinking they might still look attractive to their partner. All their negative talk turns into hostility that needs a target and the man usually is in the firing line.

As a positive, when the baby moves deep into the pelvic cavity and the head engages, ready for birth, breathing becomes bearable.

All these sensations are a good sign the finish line is very near as the baby is settling into its birth position. These changes herald in a need for complete rejuvenating rest in preparation for labor.

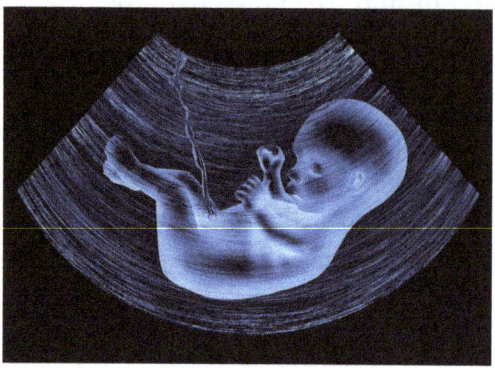

Ultrasounds

"I was so overjoyed to see my baby."

There will come a time in pregnancy where an ultrasound will be required to check on baby development. This is an easy process and nothing to really be worried about. It involves an external and internal inspection. You will need to bare your distended abdomen to the doctor who will place a freezing cold gel onto a handheld device and begin systematically moving the rounded bulge over your stomach. Special measurements of captured images are taken to establish bone and organ growth. Once finished, an internal examination is next. Taking your underpants off is the first step. Then another cold, handheld device will be gently plunged into your vagina and a new array of images will appear on the screen. To get the best images possible the medical staff making the appointment will instruct you to drink copious amounts of water before arrival. Water helps reflect the sonic waves off the organs so images of the baby are more defined.

What they don't tell you is the amount of water suggested can be far more than is really needed for great images, and the copious quantity consumed can place huge pressure on the bladder. While pregnant the bladder is extremely reactionary to becoming full, especially when you have a baby somersaulting inside adding more pressure. In most cases when attending medical appointments there is usually a long wait. Don't expect to be whisked in immediately for an ultrasound after filling up on water. A usual scenario is more likely to be you sitting on a hard chair with your bladder gradually filling up, causing a sense of urgency to urinate. Every 10 minutes the bladder fills even more without permission or opportunity to release, while your baby moves around, causing you to fear you will soon become a human Niagara Falls.

Pregnant lady after pregnant lady waddles in for their appointment, while the other women sit squirming in pain and discomfort, fearful of a sudden release. My story is similar. I struggle to convey the level of pain I went through. I broke out in a cold sweat from the agony of holding urine, trying my best to obey the rules. Fighting back tears I begged staff to allow me to release even some of the pressure. They were running terribly late. Finally after a few requests the office lady relented and said to just release half the buildup. Gulping back tears I bolted as best as any pregnant woman could to the toilet. I have no idea how I managed to hold back and only release a portion of fluid, but I did. The relief was indescribable. When examination time finally came, another ten minutes later, the doctor commented on how full my bladder was! She offered me the opportunity to release more, reassuring me she would still be able to capture the images. Hallelujah! Rejoicing in my mind I again dashed to the toilet. There was plenty of water remaining in my bladder for photos and a successful examination. All this proves to me that water consumption guidelines might not need to be so extreme.

So please, if you are extremely uncomfortable, speak up. Pregnancy and medical appointments should not have to be that hard. As a new mother you might be anxious and defer to those with appropriate training who are sometimes blinded to common sense. That was my nature back then. After such a distressing experience, I promised myself I would be more outspoken and assertive.

Please note: This story occurred when I was heavily pregnant, thus the increase in discomfort. Earlier ultrasounds were not so dramatic and waiting room times were lower.

OMG! I am so Fat, and It's Not the Baby!

"Will I ever get my body back?"

Massive distress, concern and shock can plague a woman's mind when she begins forming double chins, overflowing hips and not just a baby belly, but a huge muffin top as well. Bras no longer fit and everything becomes a squeeze. Nothing seems to stop the huge appetite or craving for fatty food to lessen the morning sickness. Before you know it, you are a horrifying 30 kilograms heavier near birth time.

Weight gain is a normal part of pregnancy. On average most women put on 15 kilograms through their pregnancy but I know of some women who gained 30 kilograms and even some who have put on a staggering 50 kilograms. The good news is the first 5 kilograms strips off quite quickly after birth as stored fluid subsides.

Then more weight-loss magic happens for most mothers through breastfeeding. If you can successfully breastfeed, then a lot of that stored fat converts after birth to the process of making milk and becomes the beautiful food for the growing baby.

It is quite amazing how week after week you can watch your

body size diminishing. Consecutive births may have slower weight loss. The biggest concern is for those women who really struggle to breastfeed and end up giving up due to either the body's inability to produce milk, nipple problems, or from emotional stress. Weight loss becomes tougher after breastfeeding is finished and depression creeps in when a mother thinks her weight will no longer return to normal. This, combined with issues surrounding a sense of failure to nurture and feed her baby, can create a toxic formula. Post-natal depression can take hold.

I suggest any woman who is really struggling with weight gain should do whatever she can to keep milk production high. Hire a lactation expressing machine as it's much easier to use than a handheld device. Best advice: just keep that milk flowing. Your self image and depression avoidance depends on this. Sadly there are always those women who cannot make milk or express successfully. Less criticism from other women, mothers and mothers-in-law can go a long way in helping them adjust to their new life and accept the weight gain as part of the baby journey. It can really take time to accept your body changes, so take it easy on yourself.

Frantic Cooking or Cleaning

"I can't stop cleaning!"

"I have already cleaned the baby clothes but now I am doing it again."

"I have turned into a germ freak!"

"What is wrong with me?

At the last minute, the 'nesting instinct' can take control. Sudden rushes of energy result in obsessive, frantic cooking, cleaning, scrubbing, or rewashing baby clothes, driving you to complete the tasks even in the middle of the night. Partners are baffled and don't want to comply with your haranguing to help and 'get with the program.' This is just another insane twist in an already taxing pregnancy in his mind. Little does he know, irrational cleaning is a common sign for early onset of labor and he should be ready for action.

You might not feel any changes in your body by way of pain or muscle contractions, but your amazing body intuition has recognized the subtle signs of hormone release already occurring, and your behavior will reflect this in making last minute preparations for the safety of your child. Your biological clock is on auto-pilot and no amount of rational intervention will prevent you from rechecking all your preparations. The nest must be ready on time.

Sometimes earlier in pregnancy you might have gone through a similar preparation phase, yet this time it feels more like an emergency. Logically it makes no sense at all to redo all your previous hard work. However, the act of cleaning can help with mental preparation and internal focus. It is important to not tire yourself from this energy expenditure, as you will need all the reserves at your disposal for birthing. Another warning can be diarrhea episodes the day before in an attempt to eliminate all fecal matter, minimizing physical energy going into other biological processes. Your body has an intelligence of its own as it moves through this beautiful stage of preparedness.

It's time to get excited. Your baby is nearly here and the long wait over!

{ 2 }

Physical and Mental Preparation

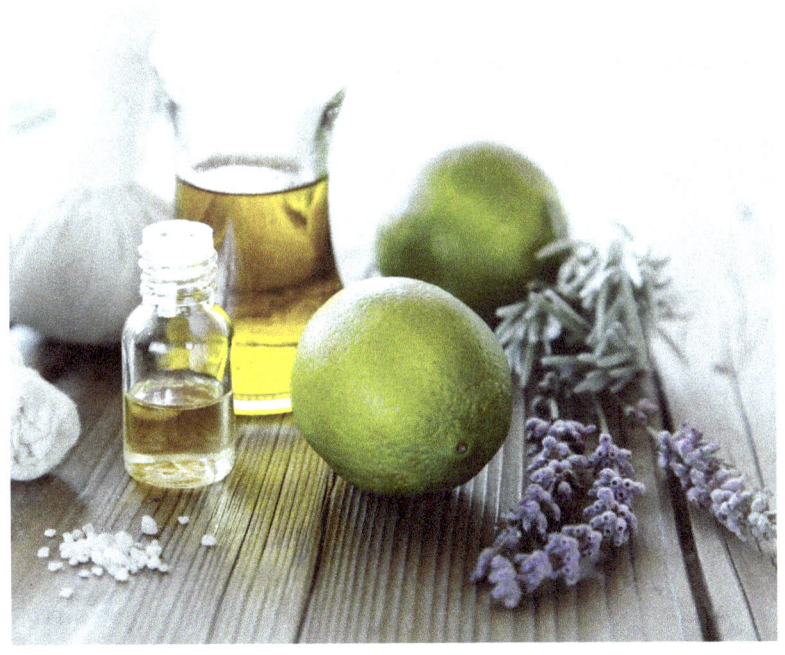

Natural Therapy Preparation Before Birth

As a natural therapist it is obvious for me to recommend some remedies that I believe can enhance your birth experience and beyond. Knowledge of natural remedies and the wisdom to take health into my own hands has really helped me as a mother feel empowered to care for my family. Our two sons have enjoyed great health with only rare situations requiring medical intervention. If I had not been a therapist myself, I would have sought out a whole array of allied health professionals to support me on my journey through motherhood. I encourage you to do the same.

There are some great natural remedies that can help you prepare for birth and in the after care of your body. Here are some remedies many women have successfully used that you might like to try. Please be aware that with remedies of any kind based on medical or naturopathic philosophy, there could be side effects and you should consult professional practitioners before going ahead.

Red Raspberry Leaf Tea or Tablets

This herb is used for strengthening and toning the uterus muscles. It's known to accelerate the birth time with less pain. Also known to shrink the uterus, after birth back to its former glory in a short time. These are currently available through health food stores, qualified naturopaths or herbalists, or sometimes through a pharmacy. Some women only take the tea in the last week of pregnancy and report great results. Others take it progressively, with greater frequency through the second and third trimesters.

I first heard about this remedy from a lady who gave birth to twins. She took raspberry leaf tea in the first and second trimester and happily gave birth to both babies in one hour after labor began. This was her second time in birthing so it was normal that labor occurred more quickly. With multiple births, babies are usually smaller, but her babies were still six pounds each.

Thrilled to hear this incredible account I began the tea at seven months, drinking three cups a day. My first son was born with no complications within four hours. My second son was born in three hours. With my second son I had taken raspberry leaf tea from the start of the second trimester. The midwives and nurses commented with surprise at how quickly the uterus muscle contracted back to acceptable hospital discharge levels by the second day.

I am aware that more doctors now mention this tea to their pregnant patients. Vets often suggest to farm animal owners to feed their pregnant mothers raspberry leaves to assist with good delivery and speedy recovery.

Homeopathic Arnica Tablets or Drops

Homeopathic arnica tablets are great to take just before and after the birth. Since the 1500s it has been a treatment for bruising and known to accelerate healing of injuries, muscle strain, sprains, rheumatic pain, and inflammation caused by fractures. It's also great on insect stings. A must have in any home first aid kit.

In relation to pregnancy and after birth care, the cream is great for dealing with localized back and stomach pain. The homeopathic drops are great for easing whole body discomfort associated with birth. When in recovery all the muscles in your body feel battered and bruised. During labor, muscles you didn't realize you even had work overtime to manage the miraculous feat of birth.

Women having caesarians gain the greatest benefits from homeopathic arnica drops or tablets. Due to the increased healing potential activated with arnica use, a woman who has been cut can move about sooner and with less body pain and discomfort than she might otherwise experience. When you are a new mum, the last thing you want is to become bedridden, barely able to lift yourself off the bed to begin breastfeeding. I have spoken with nurses about the amazing speed of recovery they had witnessed from women who used arnica.

Arnica drops can be placed in cold or warm water for after birth compresses around the anus and vagina to ease swelling and discomfort. Do not use directly on tears, episiotomy sites, or on abrasions on the vaginal tissue. To assist with speedy healing, place in the local area but not on the open wounds.

CAUTION: Do not place arnica directly on any open wounds. You will notice I have made special reference to homeopathic formulations and not the raw herb. Arnica in its *raw herbal state* can cause side effects, and ingestion is not suggested while pregnant and breastfeeding. To understand how homeopathic formulations are created seek out a qualified homeopath.

Pure 100% Essential Lavender Oil

Lavender is a natural antibiotic and can kill a variety of germs and bacteria in a safe and effective way. It's known to lessen fevers and create a calming mood when placed in bath water and has a wonderful aroma. Its antibacterial properties can help prevent infections from cracked nipples or onset of mastitis.

Lavender should only be used immediately after feeding as the smell might repel your baby from nipple attachment. Wash the breast and nipple area thoroughly before breastfeeding attempts. This oil must be 100 percent pure for its therapeutic value and skin safety. Oils made for burners often contain chemicals and substitutes, making them toxic to you and the unborn child. All essential oils should be mixed with a carrier oil such as almond, apricot kernel oil, avocado, grapeseed, olive oils and wheat germ to dilute the potency and ease application

CAUTION; Essential oils carry a strong aroma and some asthmatics react to them. Babies with undeveloped lungs might also find aromas difficult to deal with.

Other home uses:
- Treat earaches early and avoid out of control infections. Place on the earlobe, not in the ear canal.
- Sore throats – Rub the diluted oil onto the neck in the throat area. Doing this early when the sore throat first begins often prevents the onset of colds or the throat worsening.
- Apply to the chest to improve speed of recovery of coughs and chest infections.
- Apply to infected cuticles.
- Streptococcus infections can be healed with consistent use of the oil. Apply every couple of hours. Miraculously, in most cases, you can watch the infection recede and heal. If changes are not noted in the first 24 hours, seek medical advice.
- Calm sleeping by placing diluted drops onto the chest so the fragrance drifts to the nostrils or adding a few drops to bath water for a calmative effect.
- The calming effect of the oil can also assist with lowering body temperature.

Lavender oil is not just a great remedy for birth, it is another essential remedy for your home first aid kit. My family would not live without it.

Qualified aromatherapists suggest great caution around essential oil use for babies under three months. If used one drop would be maximum.

Wise Hospital Bag

Enemas: Not essential but very useful.
An enema kit, which comprises sterilized warm water, a hose, and an applicator, is a useful device to have on hand. In your prenatal classes you should learn how the pressure exerted on the

bowel can be tremendous as the baby's head squeezes through the tight space.

So if fecal matter is trapped in the lower bowel area, it's not unusual to pass bowel motions at the time of birth. Those looking on might assume your child is being born with a mucky looking hairdo.

When hearing about this prior to labor I was horrified and anxious. At the time I was not someone who liked to talk about anal waste and other body behavior. So of course I was mortified to think that my partner might see not only the baby coming out but all my other internal body wastes at the same time. So I packed a home enema kit into my hospital bag, determined to use it before labor began in earnest and to have it ready for recovery in the ward.

If you prefer not to use an enema, don't be alarmed. The body has an amazing intelligence of its own. You will usually experience urgent signals from the body before going into a high level of labor and the body will naturally want to purge itself of any unwanted pressure. (This should not be confused with the sensations that come with the bearing down phase of labor referred to later in this book.)

As a side note, some women even vomit before or during labor, thus eliminating the discomfort of undigested food remaining in the digestive tract.

Enemas after birth

Have you ever considered that after birthing you would have a difficulty in passing bowel motions? It's shockingly painful. You don't know if you should push or hold back. The pain can make you terrified of breaking or tearing stitches, or you try to hold back and not allow yourself to go to the toilet. Bowel motions have a habit of building up and solidifying, making it impossible to expel. It has to come out some time and the longer you wait the worse it will be. This is a concern, especially when people tell you of the extreme pain they experienced when passing a bowel motion the size of an orange.

After giving birth, bruising and damage can cause internal shock, resulting in the bowel action shutting down. This can be medically dangerous, so you will notice nursing staff asking about the comings and goings of fecal matter and urine. It's important to know that your body is recovering appropriately. In the ward it was quite normal for nurses to offer laxatives to some of the women.

Being forewarned, I decided to take control of my bowel actions with the help of an enema I was able to pass bowel motions successfully with little pain or discomfort. I would not have to face the fear and embarrassment of asking for laxatives and showing my weakness to the other mothers. It's funny really, the way we think as young women. We want to be seen as capable experts and not show our weaknesses. We can really put ourselves through a lot of unnecessary emotional trauma because of our attitudes. Even to the point of not asking for help when we should be screaming from the rooftops.

Paper Underwear

Paper underwear is a great invention. You can now avoid sending your partner home with blood-soaked undergarments, eliminating your mortification and his embarrassment. For that reason paper underwear is an essential item on your list of hospital bag items. These can usually be found at pharmacies. Sometimes bleeding afterwards can be intense so having emergency backups can really take the tension from your new role as mother. You can smile with confidence knowing that even though you might be running out of briefs, you do not have to cope with well-meaning mothers-in-law, moms or partners grabbing at the dirty clothing bag, determined to do a good deed. Most women like to keep that kind of body functioning private. This way handing over the bag with thanks is easy, knowing that no revealing underwear will have to be washed. Modesty saved by the paper underpants.

As an alternative, throw out all the underwear you bring to the hospital as they are often damaged with stains due to different discharges throughout the pregnancy. Start your new underwear wardrobe after birth bleeding has stopped.

Massage or TENS Machine for Labor

In prenatal classes, massage is often mentioned as a useful calming, pain relief alternative. I cannot encourage your support person enough to offer this support to you. Pain will decrease quite significantly by using specific pressure points on the lower back, followed by massage. In the absence of a support person, some hospitals may have small TENS machines (Transcutaneous electrical nerve stimulation) available for hire that can be used to great effect. If you hire this small machine, make sure it stays in the hospital bag for your important day.

Extra Food in Hospital

Organize for your partner or family members to bring some extra food or fruit into hospital. Ravenous hunger and thirst become your nightly companions when breastfeeding. Alternatively, order more food from the hospital menu than you would normally need in your evening meal, such as packed sandwiches. When waking up all through the night for feedings, hunger pangs can overtake and it will feel like an eternity before breakfast arrives.

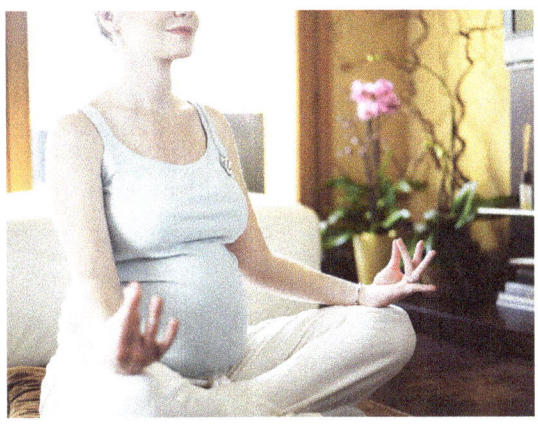

Meditation

"I am so scared. I need help."

Women who want to maintain mental and emotional focus during the birthing process should seriously think of learning some simple meditation and breathing techniques. True meditation takes quite a lot of practice and time, so I suggest for readers who are new to the meditation process to concentrate on using controlled breathing as an effective pain management regime.

In some prenatal classes breathing techniques are introduced. In the movies, rapid, raspy breathing techniques are shown and were popular in past generations. These techniques are now not frequently taught or considered a priority. The decision to not learn panting in classes might seem fine at the time, but when you are told in the middle of a huge contraction to stop pushing, you'll find it's not that simple to stop your body mid-stream. The body has a powerful impulse of its own, and this is where specific breathing techniques can help diminish the intensity of contractions and to hold back the urge to push. Holding off contractions is usually associated with medical necessity. Rapid delivery can cause tearing of the perineum. Slowing down the contractions allows more time to perform an episiotomy or allow the perineum to slowly stretch so the head and shoulders can pass through without damage to the mother. Medical interventions, such as forceps delivery, turning the head or shoulders, or removing umbilical cord obstruction, may require the rapid breathing method.

Slow breathing associated with meditation or yoga practice helps the mother to remain calm and focused, and internalizes the energy required to continue with labor. Mind you, labor will happen either way. I believe you can choose an easy or a hard way. For some women, no matter which way you choose, you may still have to deal with great trauma or an assisted birth. As an example, when I was in labor and was experiencing quite advanced pain, I found that when I remained completely focused on my slow meditative breathing, I coped with very minimal pain. As soon as I lost focus and allowed my fear to invade the process, the next contraction was terrifyingly painful! I could not believe the difference in pain levels between my disciplined mind and focus on breathing, to that of when I allowed my mind to think about what was happening in my immediate surroundings.

When you discipline thoughts and breathing, your mind is transported into a slightly altered space, ultimately lessening connections to your physical body workings. It is a great pain relief process. To establish an effective focus, choose a fixed position and avoid moving around. For some women, moving around is the only solution to discomfort and this advice may become irrelevant. Women who are established in breath work or meditation have an increased capacity to move around without losing focus.

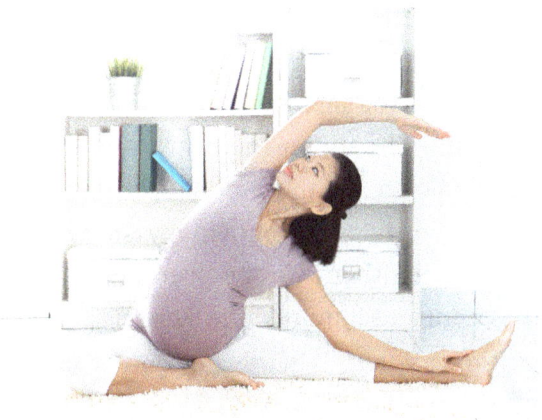

Breathing Method

Yoga or meditation breathing is quite different to the way most people breathe normally. When a baby is first born they breathe deep into the abdomen and then fill up the lungs. This is yoga breathing. Try it and see how differently we breathe. We have grown up and forgotten how to breathe with depth. Women must break the habit of sucking in their stomachs so they look slimmer. Breathing in this manner lessens the full usage of lung capacity.

Step One

Expel all the air out of your lungs and then take a deep breath in. Air taken in must first fill your abdomen, then slowly rise to fill the lower lung area and then the upper lung. You will notice that the inward breath expands the whole stomach region and causes it to distend and enlarge.

Step Two

When you are ready to expel the air, all air must leave the lung and abdomen area. You must feel the stomach falling flat and going closer to the spine. Due to expelling the air so effectively, you will feel ready to fill up again to capacity.

This breathing method is fantastic not only for birth but for health in general. If you practice these techniques while pregnant, the baby will benefit. You take in more oxygen for the blood, and the deflation of air in the abdomen pushes on the diaphragm; this acts like a pump to circulate the lymphatic fluid around the body. This system is responsible for removing waste products from the blood and eliminating them via the liver. It is directly related to the immune system and fluid retention or release.

Hypno-Birthing

"Can I be hypnotized to help get through the labor pain?"

A natural birthing alternative is hypno-birthing. This is not a new idea but it does blend more recent knowledge of hypnosis with older styles of focused thoughts and breathing techniques. With this therapy you can create prerecorded suggestions from one-on-one sessions, and bring them into the birthing suite.

Hypno-birthing uses a combination of gentle, focused breathing techniques along with self-hypnosis techniques to encourage relaxation throughout the birth process, giving way to an easier birth with less pain and anxiety. Hypnosis is at the core of therapy for couples who go to a qualified hypnotherapist for familiarization sessions. Any real birth concerns, fears or anxieties can be effectively dealt with on a one-to-one basis in progressive sessions. The therapist might choose to make a series of home recordings to use in self-hypnosis. Nearing the end of the pregnancy there will be a recording of one specific process incorporating relaxation imagery and directions to concentrate on the breath, just as you will have practiced in all the other sessions with the practitioner.

Hypnosis differs from meditation through the use of encoding the subconscious to act on a word trigger, and suggestions to assist the mind in reclaiming inner calm and mental balance. Many women find this to be a powerful tool in their birthing arsenal.

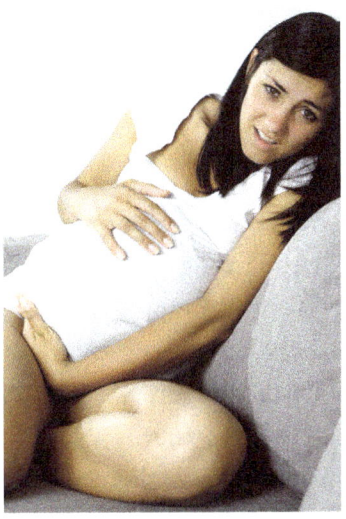

Braxton Hicks Contractions

"What are the contractions I have from time to time in my early pregnancy?"

Nature is remarkable. Prior to birth the body can move through a series of contractions mimicking the labor state. These abdominal gripping muscle spasms are called "Braxton Hicks" contractions and can occur at any time in the pregnancy. They are more commonly felt in the last trimester as a preparation and toning of the uterine muscles. However, I experienced them at the beginning of my second trimester and know of other women who also started early. They can be quite extreme and alarming when they occur, often causing panicked thoughts of the baby coming early.

Stay calm and just time your contractions. If they remain

constant and occur in an even sequence, medical supervision should be sought. If, however, you experience these uncomfortable sensations and pain for only a few contractions before releasing, just breathe easy and know the body is preparing through practice.

The Braxton Hicks sensations can be mild fluttery tightness over the abdomen area (not to be confused with baby movements). Many women I have spoken to experienced quite severe pain that would grip the insides intensely. I also experienced this pain—sometimes the gripping sensations would become extremely strong and my whole abdomen would tighten in a continuous vice-like grip. Timing some of these sensations, I noted they lasted up to forty-five minutes without reprieve. My breathing techniques came in handy, as did sitting in strange positions in an attempt to take the pressure off.

If it occurs while your partner is around, you might also have to try to calm them and instruct them to keep an eye on the clock. Alert them that an emergency exit may be required—and no, they cannot go and have another beer or pop down to the pub! Some men actually ask this!

If these sensations frighten or alarm you, and you feel they might be happening too often, it does no harm to arrange a checkup with your midwife or doctor. Better to be safe and informed.

Some women never experience the Braxton Hicks sensations, so they miss out on that early insight of a real labor situation. It is for this reason I have included the next section of exercises to help you have some idea of what to expect.

Body awareness exercise to familiarize yourself to Braxton Hicks contractions and early labor

This next exercise in body observation may seem a little unorthodox but it really is quite insightful for relieving pre-labor anxiety and the Braxton Hicks contraction phenomena. The bowel function is going to be the focal point. Anyone who has had extreme diarrhea would have felt the bowel muscles gripping and contracting just before fecal matter is expelled from the body. The sensations of an imminent explosive bowel movement are very similar to the sensations that grip the abdomen with the onset of Braxton Hicks contractions. If you want to know what they can feel like, imagine you are on the toilet and diarrhea is imminent.

Imagine sitting buckled over the seat staring at the floor. You can feel the rise and fall of sensations washing over you. The pain at times increases or locks on as you sit wondering when relief and release will occur. The pain is building up with intensity but nothing seems to be moving. By now the body is heating up and perspiration begins to bead on the brow. The whole body wants to push but still nothing occurs while the stomach gradually feels nauseous as pressure intensifies.

Finally after much panting and gripping the abdomen, relief is at hand. Blissful sensations flow over the body as muscles relax and normalize again. But don't be tricked; you're not finished yet! Just when you're about to leave, another urge overwhelms, pants are ripped to the ground, and again the diarrhea dance takes hold. It's a weird comparison to explain a Braxton Hicks experience, yet it's very effective. So as you can see, both men and women can have an insight into what Braxton Hicks can feel like. No one misses out!

Pre-Labor Visualizations and Exercises

"What does labor feel like? How can I prepare myself?"

Labor pains can feel similar to Braxton Hicks contractions, but the lead-up is quite different. It is usually slower and less intense, slowly building up into a crescendo. To understand your body and its muscle movements, it helps if you focus attention on your body's activity. Get to know your body and its actions in intimate detail. Breathe and be aware of your bodily functions and how each area feels. Become sensitive to the body's every activity. Many liken the early stages of labor to bad period pains that slowly intensify over time. The time between each episode of pain will also shorten. It is also quite common for back pain to be present.

There is a way to experience the sensations of labor in a milder form. It is similar in technique to the Braxton Hicks and again uses bowel movements as a focus. I credit this approach to a wise lady who passed it onto me. She instructed me to observe every bowel motion so I understood the intelligence of the body by feeling for the different sensations within the bowel and abdomen while defecating. The critical point to her instruction was to become aware that the body will remove fecal matter without the need for our interference.

After listening to her I began practicing the exercises immediately. My reward was lower anxiety and a trust in my body's intelligence during the birthing process. I was amazed to discover that when entering labor my body commanded all the muscles to push without my mind being engaged in the process. I was able to lie back and just focus on the breathing. The only time my mind was activated to even think of pushing and assisting birth was near the end when the nurses instructed. The rest of the time my body did the work while my mind relaxed into rhythmic breathing.

I pass this technique on to you.

Visualization

Imagine not having a bowel movement for a couple of days. This is very easy to imagine when pregnant, since constipation seems to go hand in hand with the experience. Bowel motions use the same muscles as the uterus muscles. They are called smooth muscles and are part of the autonomic nervous system—they do not require a mental connection to contract the muscle. These similarities mean you can actually practice a technique that provides insight and mental preparation for labor. The technique is practiced while sitting on the toilet and in the process of defecating. You will discover that birthing has a resemblance to defecating, and you can develop skills for a calm breathing method while in labor.

When sitting on a toilet, begin yoga breathing and observe your body. Feel the rise and fall of muscle sensations, but Do Not Push. Just observe and breathe. Feel the small movements within the abdomen. This could feel like an unusual pressure building up of its own accord. You have no control over these sensations; they arise automatically, as the body has its own intelligence.

Mimicking Early Labor

As the pressure builds, calm those busy thoughts and focus your mind awareness upon your body and the sensations arising within. When your body is ready to perform a bowel movement, you will feel a rise in pressure, with muscles gently beginning to grip the internal abdominal region. These sensations mean that you must follow the urge to defecate. Instead of being active in the process and trying to push to speed the process up, just sit, breathe, and observe. As you do this, you will notice that without any effort on your part the abdomen will grip tight. When it does, just keep your breathing even and focused; eventually the gripping hold will release. After a pause, you will feel it again—the abdomen squeezes and contracts. Within the contraction you might feel a barely perceptible movement of the feces. If you keep breathing through the sensation, you will discover there is no need to push. It does it magically on its own.

Mimicking the Active Phase of Labor

If you keep observing the gripping, squeezing sensation within the abdomen you'll be aware of how the sensations rise and fall in regular intervals. This is how early labor contractions will feel, only they will gradually become more intense. The trick is to keep breathing through the gripping sensation with a calm mind and allow the body to do what it knows best. With each bowel contraction the urgency intensifies as the fecal matter progressively enters into the lower passage, ready to be expelled. You become acutely aware of the size of the mass trying to come out. This is how the head will feel, but it's more like a bowling ball needing to be expelled and the whole pelvis will yawn, open unable to stop itself.

Mimicking the Bearing Down Pushing Phase, Crowning and Birth

When the fecal matter is close to exiting, the anus stretches to capacity and you will feel your whole body gathering an inner energetic momentum. Every muscle is summoned, giving way to last-minute waves of pushing until the fecal matter explodes out of you. It is only then that you will feel a pause in the pushing sensations. This is just like the birth of the head, but you'll still have the shoulders to go. Another burst of pushing sensations follows. More fecal matter expels, and this is likened to the shoulder of the baby freeing up, and then the whole body slides out.

Mimicking Placental Birth

Placental birth is delayed as your body has minute contractions to recover from the major birth. This also occurs with the last parts of a bowel motion. Small contractions build up until the last part is expelled and then you know you are done.

My Apologies for the Gross Comparisons

I know this seems an incredibly gross way to explain the process of labor, and the eventual birth of your long awaited child. For me to go as far as drawing a parallel to those magic moments of welcoming your new child into the world and comparing it to a bowel motion can be offensive. Please understand this visualization technique is more about understanding the muscle actions that are taking place, with special emphasis on how it might feel as a direct experience and as a way to steady your mind and emotions when real labor begins.

CAUTION: If you continue to force out bowel movements when pregnant, there is a risk of damaging the blood vessels in the anus. This can cause hemorrhoids that are very uncomfortable. As I mentioned earlier, women during pregnancy after giving birth are at a high risk of this occurring anyway. There is no reason to increase the risk by being in a hurry. Use this time to be mindful. Perhaps men have already discovered the art of toilet mindfulness; this would explain the extreme length of time they like to sit in the cubicle. Now it's the women's turn.

Pain Tolerance

"I am so anxious, I don't know if I can deal with the pain."

One of the hardest predictors is your coping ability through labor. Everyone has a different pain tolerance and because of this many irregularities in a couple's communication might arise. Pain can cause some crazy emotional states along with other physical reactions. A woman with high pain tolerance might not speak up until a problem that could have been averted is well and truly advanced and the pain eventually hits their threshold. They seem to push through amazing levels of pain and discomfort. Then there is the woman who appears as though she has a high pain tolerance, only she is so terrified to be a problem to other people she resorts to using sheer willpower to not ask for help. Low pain tolerance can be so extreme that upon the first hint of pain this woman is quick to become shaky, faint or cry at a moment's notice.

These huge discrepancies make it difficult for partners to read the true situation as it unfolds. If the woman is not panicking and seems relaxed, it might not seem as though advanced labor has begun. Driving to the hospital might be dangerously delayed, causing a car birth. The non-complainer could be bleeding, yet does not like to be a bother, so leaves the alert until last minute. In the meantime she is hoping someone can read her mind and realize she desperately needs support and medical attention. Then there is the low pain threshold woman, who goes into multiple panics day after day demanding a hospital visit when only experiencing Braxton Hicks. She might be self-imposed bed-bound, as she cannot even cope with the abdominal discomfort of carrying a child. All these scenarios are potential annoyances for partners trying their utmost to read the situations and provide adequate and relevant support and action. They also provide fertile soil for a woman to begin angering and blaming as she vents through her pain.

This misreading a woman's coping mechanism does not end with the partner. Hospital staff will also become confused and potentially misread vital signs. It is up to the support person to help them understand the personality type they are dealing with to better enable them to provide effective and precise care.

If you are not sure what type of personality you have in relation to pain then as a general guide the way you handle normal pain events will become indicative in how labor will affect you. Having said that, never underestimate the power of instinct; it has the power to keep a person completely focused and coping until after the birth, then old habits will reappear.

So far I have only addressed the reactions of women in pain during labor. Think about your partner: how do they handle pain and blood in normal situations? There is a good chance that all the best intentions and expectations of providing and receiving support could fly out the window. Fainting, gagging partners are common. Even strong high pain threshold partners might only manage pain well for themselves yet when faced with a partner in pain or gruesome blood events, they could be triggered into a whole different state.

It is vitally important you understand the limitations each of you have, especially in relation to pain.

Support, what does that mean?

"I worry that my partner might not be able to cope."

"What if my partner doesn't make it to the hospital and I am all alone?"

Micro-managing the birth experience is a great starting point, but have you discussed what to do, or how you will manage situations that are not in your plans? It's great to discuss with your partner all your hopes for the birth and how it will eventuate; however, expect most of your birth plans and explanations to fall on deaf ears. When a woman is pregnant, it is really hard for the man to even connect to the idea that out of her huge bugling belly, a baby will emerge. Not only is it incomprehensible, but for them to even imagine the birth scene and how they will feel when faced with blood, sounds of pain, medical examinations and all the confusion to come, is a mere impossibility. So men often switch off their minds to all the information you give them and filter out other people's birth stories. Men never really explain to each other how the birth of the their child affected them, so your male partner might not feel it's important to listen appropriately to your needs until it's too late.

Avoid long lists. Men generally take action with practical requests and go into domestic deafness when talking about lighting, music, crystals and massage oils. Don't confuse his brain otherwise he will shut off from all of your plans. Define the most important features that must be included in the birth process. If you do not want pain relief, try to drum that into your partner's mind. When faced with howling screams he may demand they give you something, anything to make the noise stop. Even when you scream for it he will more likely be convinced you really want the drugs instead of talking you through the pain. He will want to crash tackle a staff member to the ground to help his partner not have to go through the torture he is witnessing.

When it comes to medical interventions, with after birth care, vaccinations, needles, washing the baby or stitching the torn perineum, you need to really emphasize the importance of your partner helping you, stick to the prearranged birth plan. If he knows how important this is to you he might be able to find the confidence to speak up to medical personnel and move through his own feelings of confusion and the fear of challenging authority.

In this instance, in a strange and warped way, you are the lucky one. There is no choice but to birth the baby. No turning back. So when you are faced with the sheer magnitude of the birthing event you have to proceed with labor in any way it presents. Control is no longer in your hands so a support person needs to be equipped to handle situations that might arise. They will also need to be given permission to leave the birth area for a break when their own anxiety takes over and they feel overwhelmed.

For this reason many women choose a female relative who has already given birth herself, or a 'Doula' (birth attendant) to be the eyes and ears for you. They intimately know the different stages your body is going through and can talk and encourage you with minimal fuss and anxiety. In fact, they can also explain to your partner what is happening because by then, he is all ears to understand the perplexing situation he has found himself in.

Thinking your partner will be 100% engaged and able to support in any event should be rethought. By the time he is faced with the gory reality of blood, water and pain, he is usually overwhelmed by anxiety, guilt and feeling extremely powerless. Forced to watch it all unfold and have no idea which way to turn; how to communicate with medical personnel, ensuring they follow your plan; or how to protect you from the ordeal you are going through becomes a mammoth task. Many men express their guilt over being underprepared and not listening attentively to their partner early in the pregnancy.

Special Note: The beautiful picture you have in your mind about the amazing support you will receive can often seem irrelevant once you are in the middle of birthing. You will be totally focused on the job and everyone in the birthing suite becomes a blurry bother. Do not be surprised if all the loving, fussy support from your partner becomes an insane irritation.

Examples of a partner's support or seeming lack thereof:

- While in a hospital ward waiting for my own labor to kick in properly, I saw one father constantly checking the football results as his wife sat groaning in the bed. Since she was sitting upright and looked as though she was managing ok, he thought it was fine to take off and see the game results from time to time.

Next time I saw him he had bolted from the labor suite, pale and trembling, heading outside to have a cigarette. When I asked him what he was doing, he explained in trembling tones how terrible it was in there and he couldn't cope. He was not even sure he could return.

- My husband, exhausted from a couple of hours of massaging and hovering, with the added 1am start, fell asleep on the comfortable bed by my side while I was on the verge of delivering. Fortunately for him I was not a screamer.

Other stories of women and their men include:
- A completely overwhelmed and nervous man, who could not cope with the guttural sounds erupting from his wife, desperately tried to leave the room only to be dragged back by his wife's mother.
- A man suddenly vomiting on the floor in sympathy when he saw his partner vomit.
- Men nervously patting their partner offering (to the woman ears while in labor) inane words of support.
- A husband, who had his offers of drinks and ice to his partner abruptly rejected, felt useless so he sat in the corner of the room and flash up his lap top and play games on his laptop. He did this until birth, only helping with the cord when berated by a midwife.

These stories might shock; yet once a woman has completed labor she is usually not able to completely recall where their partner actually was through the whole process. Her entire focus was inward and getting the baby out! So don't stress the small details, they become unimportant. More importantly, try not to place huge expectations and demands on how your partner must support you. This only leads to disappointment.

Oxytocin, the Love Chemical

Midwives, nursing staff and written research all report on the amazing correlation that mental and emotional attitude has on the overall birth process. Birthing mothers presenting as anxious seem to become overwhelmed by a torrent of intense pain, elongated labor, complications and assisted deliveries. Other women who remain calm and focused, have a softly spoken support person, and who breathe through the process on average have a lower incident rate of intervention or unbearable pain.

This is attributed to the presence of oxytocin hormones in the birth process. When high levels of oxytocin is released through the body, labor begins. Intervals of release continue throughout the labor. If these hormones are interrupted for any reason then the birth process can delay or stop. This could happen at any stage, potentially causing harm to the baby by distressing it. The enemy of oxytocin is adrenaline. Under extreme stress the body is activated into the fight/flight response, In effect this prepares the body to gather all the resources it has and run to safety, and in doing so shuts down all other functions until the danger has passed. This is of course the opposite behavior you need for birth.

Oxytocin release is supported and activated in environments that a female brain associates with love. Beautiful music, sounds of water, subdued lighting, soft gentle words, romance and sex all enhance oxytocin release.

Bright lights, clanging metal sounds, loud and irritated voices, tension, anxiety and above all FEAR on the other hand, activate adrenaline.

Internal and external environments all have their influence. Trying your best to create a safe space will make all the difference to your experience of birth. If plans fail then you still have the greatest calming action available, your breath.

Happy Birth Orgasms

"I could not believe birthing could have moments that felt so beautiful and connected."

Giving birth does not have to be terrible. In fact some women state they experience pleasurable orgasms during labor. This can happen multiple times, lasting on averaging up to 15 seconds. It's not often talked about because some women feel embarrassed or guilty for experiencing pleasurable sensations through birth, normally ascribed to sexual intimacy. It's sad to know they feel this way when they have no control over the outcome. Orgasms can also offer significant pain relief due to releasing endorphins and oxytocin hormones. These are the same hormones that are released with the experience of falling in love. Some couples have taken matters into their own hands and instead of hoping for spontaneous orgasm, they sexually self-stimulate as part of a pain management regime.

Debra Pascall-Bonaro became a well-known documentary maker with her controversial film *Orgasmic Birth: The Best Kept Secret*. Her documentary has created a whole new conversation around birth experiences.

Giving birth does not have to be a scary experience. Your emotional approach can make all the difference. Claim your orgasmic birth today.

Breech Position? Don't Panic, It Can be Changed

Breech position can be changed close to labor to aid in a stress-free birth. Breech is the most difficult birth position as it means the baby is laying upright presenting with their feet or bottom first and not their head. Many babies have already positioned themselves weeks before into the anterior birth position, known as the most effective position, due to the even pressure placed upon the neck of the uterus during contractions. The head helps the cervix widen due to hormones released with the added pressure. The back of the baby's head nestles nicely into the pelvic cavity and does not place heavy pressure on the mother's back. This position also allows the head to tilt as it moves through the birth canal with the smallest part of the head presenting first. If the head doesn't tilt, the experience will be similar to your own head trying to push through a turtle-neck shirt without tucking the chin under.

One in ten babies in Western cultures begin labor in the posterior position. This position can cause distressing pain in the lower back due to the skull being forced against the spinal column. Other common issues might be water breaking early, long and arduous labor with the sensation to push arising when the cervix has not dilated yet, and to top it off the baby must be turned 180 degrees for a successful birth. This can take some time and in the end you may need a forceps or suction cup (ventouse) to assist delivery.

The cause for so many Westerners experiencing breech birth is our tendency to live sedentary lives. We no longer scrub floors, work the fields, pick crops or till the soil. We have wonderful washing machines that take the back-breaking work out of thrashing clothes upon a rock. We see this as great advancement for our daily lives, yet our sisters in developing countries enjoy going into labor, regularly giving birth to babies in the anterior position. Hard-core chores done on a daily basis causes the pelvis to tilt in ways that become uncomfortable so the baby begins to move until finding the perfect fit in the pelvic cavity. That position just so happens to be the best and most comfortable for the woman during birth. Equipped with this knowledge makes it easier to change some of our habits to try to get the baby to turn before birth.

Changing the Birth Position from Breech or Posterior

Medical personnel will attempt to turn your baby when either in breech or posterior position to avoid the higher risk of caesarean. They use a technique called the External Cephalic Version (ECV), which is usually done just prior to labor or in the early onset.

As a natural therapist, part of my training is in remedial massage. Through the years I have seen countless women who have presented at the clinic with babies in breech position. By developing a simple turning procedure using massage and positioning techniques the baby is encouraged to move into the correct birth position. Special training is not required, so it's fine for other people to try it. I have used this skill countless times to facilitate the baby to roll over. This technique is classified as a spontaneous turning event known as SCV, (spontaneous cephalic version)—when the baby turns of its own accord.

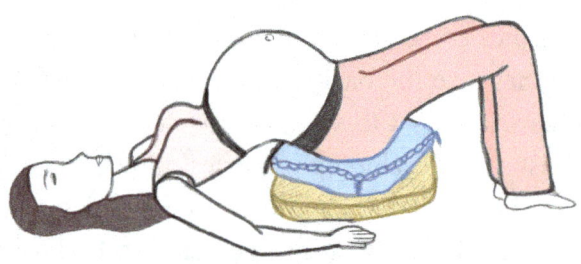

This technique is achieved by having the woman lay down on a fairly firm surface. Then place many pillows under her bottom until she is lying in a significant slant position. Gravity helps the baby fall away from the birth position and ever so slightly leaves some space for the baby to move. Now that the woman is relaxed, begin massaging the stomach, but more importantly the baby. Light fluffy movements will put the baby to sleep. This treatment needs to be more like kneading dough and pushing the baby in slow rhythmic actions, away from the pubic bone, avoiding frantic movements. The idea is if you can disrupt the baby's position a little, he or she might decide to shift and hopefully roll into position. This usually occurs hours after the massage technique has been implemented or overnight.

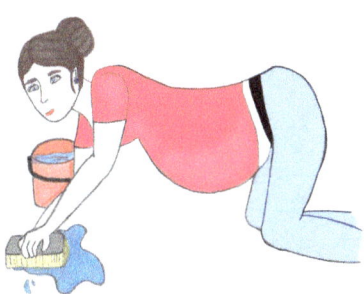

Alternatively you can use other skills in the home. The general idea is to create an environment that makes the baby uncomfortable and disengaged from either the breech position (feet first) or the posterior position—effectively you need to unsettle the baby and make them quite uncomfortable. Become more active, avoid standing all day without radically changing position, avoid lying back on recliner chairs as the pelvis tilts in the wrong direction. Follow past generational advice by scrubbing the floor, clean out low cupboards or, as some people suggest, have sex in a kneeling position. If you choose this option there is higher risk of sexual discomfort due to deep penetration. Having said that, if you are overdue it is often suggested to have sex to stimulate labor.

Don't panic if the baby doesn't move; often in early stages of labor they can still roll successfully into the best birth position.

{ 3 }

No Turning Back

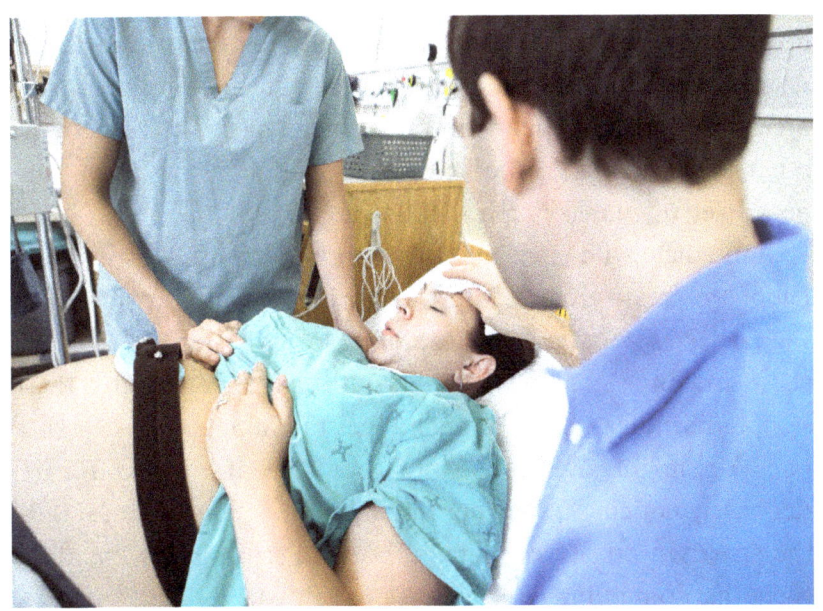

Celia Fuller

Mentally Unprepared Men

"I thought real labor meant the waters broke first."

It is important to check with your partner on his/her perception or belief about what labor looks like. Their answer will give you a fair idea about how much information through prenatal classes and books they have actually taken in. Usually their idea of birthing is quite different to the reality.

Due to the constant barrage of television shows depicting instant frenzied labor, men and women are left to believe this is how you can recognize with 100% surety that labor has begun. Another belief might be that labor does not begin until the waters break. So partners might think they have plenty of time to get other jobs done since the strong expected signs have not happened yet, often delaying hospital transport.

Immediate wild cramping pains are not the usual experience. Labor progressively creeps up, requiring watchful attention for the early signs of diarrhea, grumbling lower back pain, a bloody show, and unusual pain symptoms in the pubic bone. Often these symptoms indicate early labor and they might not be present all at once. You might have slipped into labor without you or your partner barely noticing. A partner might not take serious notice until the screaming phase or agitated hot and frustrated stage alerts them that something is wrong.

By the time obvious contractions begin you have really entered established labor and should be making your way to the hospital, unless you've chosen a home birth. When you become hot and flustered or go unusually quiet then you know you are treading on dangerous territory, and in a worst case scenario it could be a matter of minutes before the baby is actually born.

Don't delay, call the hospital or midwife and ask for guidance. Travel to the hospital as soon as you can.

'The Bloody Show' – Mucous Plug (Operculum)

When pregnant, the body forms a mucous plug that acts as a lid on the cervix, which keeps bacteria from the uterus, lessening the risk of infection and harm to the baby. At some point it will dislodge and pass painlessly out of the vagina. It might appear as mucous blobs with small amounts of blood or even look like a slug. You might notice the passing when wiping after a toilet visit, or it's naturally fallen into the toilet or left on the underpants, sometimes after medical examinations or after sex. Do not be alarmed if blood is evident, your baby is safe. Blood is usually present due to the cervix dilating and minutely tearing some tiny blood vessels as part of the process of labor preparation. The plug can come away weeks before actual birthing. Your baby remains safe in the uterus while ever the amniotic fluid remains intact. This fluid is the second layer of protection from infection. If the waters break, however, then medical support would be advised.

Breaking Water

Breaking water is an eerie experience. Contrary to belief from media footage, waters breaking in one gigantic gushing moment is not the only way to experience this event. Gentle breaking, followed by trickling or gushing intervals as you walk is also possible. It feels like copious amounts of fluid leaking from your lower half. The sensations feel as though there is far more evacuating than really is. It can be likened to a heavy period and the associated paranoia of overflow is close behind. When your waters break naturally it is a sign that labor will soon begin. This fluid comes from the placental sack which cushions the baby from external movements or sudden jolts. It also keeps the developing child in a hygienic environment free from germs or bacteria. Waters not broken before labor will either naturally break or have to be broken by medical staff to help bring the labor on. This process can be quite daunting.

A sudden rush of fluid and blood comes gushing out along with an overwhelming sense of horror when realizing that medical people are standing right in the line of fire. This experience is so far from what I would define as dainty and would be definitely in the humiliating category! Then again, most pregnancy and birth experiences are full of awkward humiliating moments so there is sure to be more to replace this one, allowing it to recede in importance.

The greatest fear for many women is the thought of her waters breaking in a public place. For those who are paranoid about this possibility it is suggested to carry a towel wherever you go. Avoiding public places can be quite normal preference nearing the end of term. This makes it difficult on the home front as partners do not comprehend the anxiety and chores still need to be done. It's not easy conveying to the man how devastating the idea is of water trickling down the legs and covering a supermarket floor, then having to get some pimply faced kid to come and mop it up. For these possible situations definitely keep a towel with you.

It is important that any breaking of the water should be reported to the maternity ward of your designated hospital. If this occurs medical staff usually prefer mothers to come to the hospital for observation. This is simply a precaution for the safety of the child. When the waters break the baby no longer exists in the sterile environment that the placental sack provides. Once the protection is broken, risk of infection becomes the concern. Staff will monitor your progress once you are safely under their observation and care.

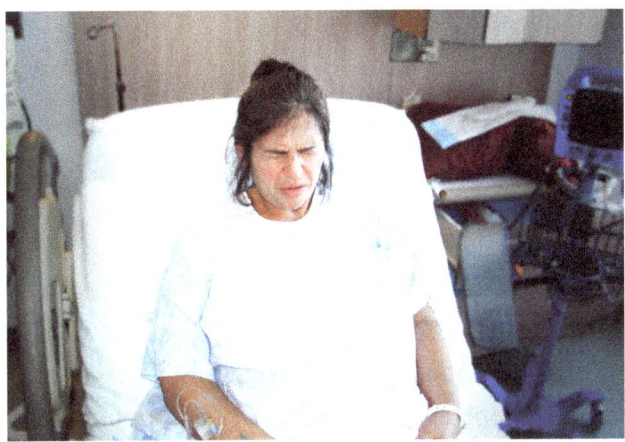

Labor Begins

Labor is varied for every woman and there are many choices around birthing preferences: no medical pain intervention, home or hospital, water or not. Labor is fraught with the best laid plans going awry, so I will not pose as an expert in this area, rather I will focus on the stages you enter and how the body can feel internally to aid in mental preparation. Labor comes in three stages: early labor, established labor (pushing and birth phase), and birth of placenta.

The First Stage

Early Phase Labor

Prior to the real labor occurring you might experience contractions, but regularity can be a little erratic, occurring every 20-30 minutes, and it can last for days or sometimes weeks.

-Pain is similar to period pain.

-You might have the mucous plug known as 'The Bloody Show' come away, with a small amount of blood showing

- experience loose bowel movements
- urge to vomit
- lower back pain
- cervix might be dilated 3-6 cm

Active Labor

When the pains become regular at ten minutes apart, you will enter a settled rhythm of an active labor. The body will become settled and focused upon birth as the outcome. The cervix will soften and thin out, preparing for the baby's head to move through.

Contractions will intensify with increased pain. The abdomen will lock into a tight hold, taking your breath away, then release, taking a pause before the next wave of pain ensues. Pauses in between are a great relief. At this stage conversations are possible. Pain will continue to intensify as the intervals between contractions shorten. When this occurs, the mind shifts and becomes vague and slightly disconnected from immediate surroundings and people. An amazing power takes over mental acuity, and it feels as though all the energy is internalizing in an amazing mind-body focus. This is a strange state and not one that is easy to convey but is a prelude to deeper, mind shattering contractions. You need to breathe with the contractions, not panic. Remember I mentioned, the more you panic the worse the pain seems.

By now the cervix will be opening wider, taking you across the threshold from active labor to a medical phrase called established labor.

- Contractions changing from 10 minutes apart to 4-5 minutes lasting 40 to 60 seconds
- Dilated up to 6-8 cm

The first stage of labor is completing, moving into the second stage. By now you might begin feeling erratic and restless.

Established Labor and Birthing – Second Stage Transition

Screaming Obscenities Stage. Cervix opens to 10cm fully dilated.

Shifting into transition is announced by sensations of overheating, annoyance, impatience or restlessness along with extreme discomfort in your bowels convincing you to use them. If hospital staff overhears comments of urgent bowel motion sensations, you will be whipped off to a birthing suite in a frenzy. It means the baby's head has begun the journey through the cervix entering into the vagina. Birth could occur anytime now, so staff will be alert. First pregnancies might remain longer in the transition phase so there is usually time to resettle into labor after travelling from home or moving from one ward to another.

Expect constant poking and probing between your legs from now on, as staff assess how dilated you are and how close actual birth will be. You could be stuck in this phase for hours waiting for the cervix to dilate sufficiently for a successful birth. The baby's heartbeat will be monitored, ensuring it is not becoming distressed. If there is any suggestion of this, a Caesarean will be seriously considered. In your vague state you may hear them speak of this.

Partners will be frantically trying to mop your sweaty brow or massage your back in an attempt to eliminate your pain and give comfort, all the while avoiding flying fists. Dependent on their resilience some might have already passed out from the graphic details or are just sleeping through the whole event. No matter what they are doing there is a high risk they will be blamed and verbally assaulted for something.

- Stronger contractions 1-2 minutes in between and lasting up to 60–90 seconds with intense peaks
  - Vagina will feel some burning due to stretching
  - Nausea or vomiting, shaking cramps
  - Pressure in the bottom
  - Urge to push

Special Note: Not all women scream frantically or abuse their partners. There are many women who settle into a rhythm, remain calm, make no fuss, breathe deeply and groan. If you keep practicing the breathing techniques this can be your experience too.

What does transition feel like?

It is at the stage that all your plans for the birth start to derail. Allow yourself to become disengaged to your surroundings and surrender to the primal power of labor, thinking about the baby and the extreme process it has to go through.

Pain starts to rip you apart; your mind screams in horror, not believing it will survive the journey. There are stories abound of women screaming, throwing punches and demanding for everyone to make it stop. The pain is enough for any woman to rethink the idea of having a natural birth without pain relief. Martyrdom goes out the window. By this stage it is already too late for most pain relief interventions; you are committed and yelling/screaming will only make it worse.

It's here you must remember to breathe! Observe the body sensations and breathe through the pain. Screaming tenses you up. If you become fearful of the pain and believe you can't cope, you will find the pain increases by 90%. Your mind becomes the enemy. When you tense up the pain becomes mind blowing.

You must begin to settle and trust those breathing exercises and let the mind focus. It's at this stage, you will wish you listened more and practiced more. When in pain, it is not automatic to breathe through the pain. The natural fight/flight response has you feeling like you want to run as far away as possible or fight with screaming, blaming words. More settled mothers might start to feel deep, powerful groans and moans erupting. With focused breath and deep groans you can seamlessly move into the next stage of needing to push.

SPECIAL NOTE TO MEN: If it looks like everything is going wrong, it's really going right. When your partner starts saying she cannot do this anymore, this is your indicator the transition phase has been entered. It's not long now!

Get the baby out! Pushing

Suddenly a quietness of the spirit enters your space as the body pauses and summons every ounce of energy for this next phase.

If you thought your contractions were strong before, then the power housed within your own body will shock and amaze. By now your mind does not belong to you. When it's time to push, don't worry too much because the body's intelligence takes over and pushing starts without you even having to try. By now your mind can only watch what happens as the body takes over and gets the job done.

The good news is labor is nearly over!

Every muscle and fiber of your body bears its force towards the baby to assist in its progression through the birth canal and out into the world. It's important at this stage to breathe calmly and remain alert to any instructions from nursing staff. Your body is doing all the pushing but when the head crowns or the baby has to be turned, or the cord is presenting incorrectly, the doctor or midwife will tell you to stop pushing. When they instruct you in this way, you might be inclined to panic because you know your mind has not been telling your body to push, your body has been on autopilot. So you would think it's impossible, but you can actually slow the process down by changing your breathing. Short quick panting-like breaths will slightly interrupt the full force of the pushing sensations. This can give just enough time for maternity staff to attend to the baby. Slowing the birth process down can mean the difference between tearing badly or an episiotomy (surgical cut). It can also help staff adjust the baby's exit position. Whatever you do, just keep panting until they tell you to push hard. That's when you have to use the full force of your will, mind and muscles to push even harder, until your baby is born.

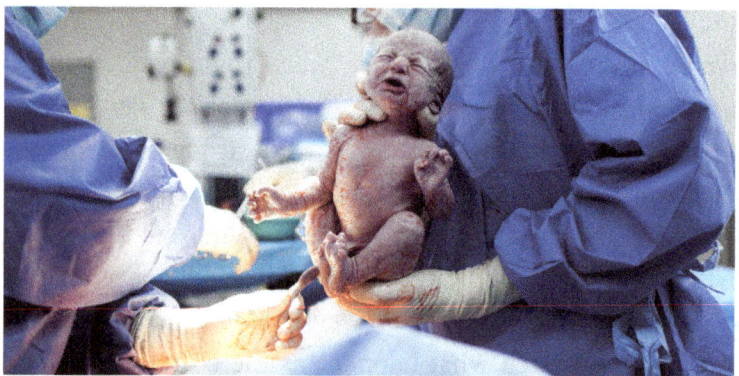

Crowning

At first, the crown of the head appears, remaining in that position for a few more pushes. Gathering momentum, contractions contort to exert extreme downward pressure in order to push the baby's head out through the tight vaginal opening.

(Episiotomy or tearing occurs at this stage). Internally there is an overriding sense of relief after birthing the head along with searing pain or heat in the vagina. With the head safely out the body needs to attend to birthing the shoulders. The next contraction exerts another huge push to free shoulders up and the rest of the baby will rapidly slip out, all wet, bloody and slimy. Your whole body will go into a relaxation pause as silence fills the room only to be broken by the reassuring wails of your baby's cry. This sudden burst of sound guarantees an inhalation of oxygen filling the lungs of your newborn child. Frantic activity from the staff will have the baby's cord cut and baby placed on your belly.

Note: With birth comes a lot of blood and fluid, and sometimes fecal matter is forced out from the severe strain. You may not be aware of this as your full concentration is on pushing but a partner may have access to the full visual and become a little faint. All of this is normal.

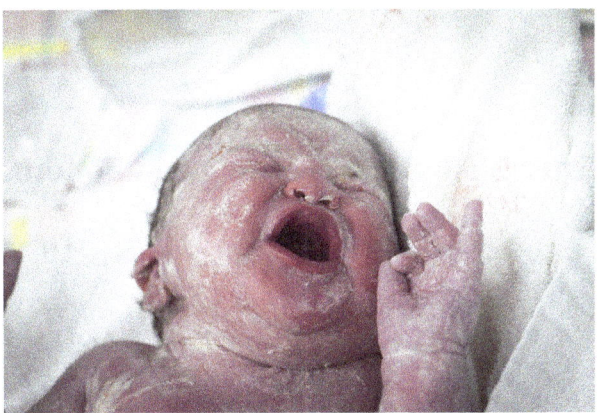

When the baby is placed upon you or wrapped up, it will look slightly distorted, covered in wax. This substance has been a protector while in utero and remains a great barrier from bacteria as the newborn adjusts to the physical world. In the past, babies used to be washed immediately. These days nursing staff encourage leaving washing for a couple of days. You may also notice your baby has a distorted head or face. Don't panic; the head will adjust to a normal shape once their cranial bones move and shift into place. It's not easy for a baby's head to be squeezed through such a small space so the cranial bone miraculously shifts to help with birthing.

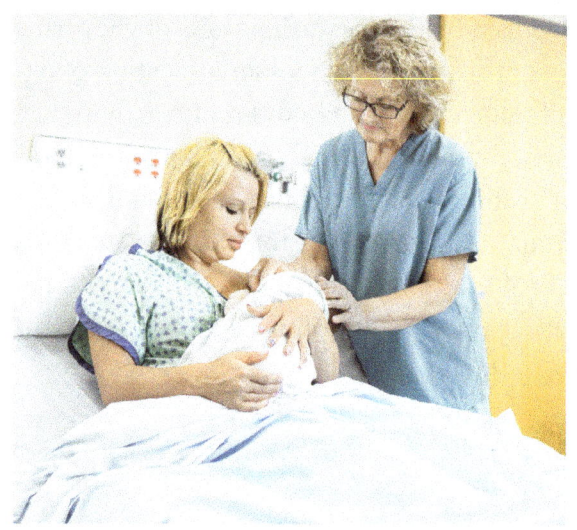

After Birth Breast Feeding and Bonding

"He bit me! No one told me it hurts!"

"What is wrong with me? I did not feel instant love for my baby."

Feeding

Straight after the birth, if your baby is in a healthy state a nurse will encourage you to breastfeed. This immediate feed is instigated for two reasons. Firstly, to process the colostrum known as the fore milk into their body's system as soon as possible. The colostrum is full of antibodies that strengthen the immune system and provides an immediate barrier to the bacteria and germs they will now come into contact with. Secondly, contractions are stimulated to encourage the birth of the placenta. Yes that's right, labor has not finished yet!

Babies bite! If you have been led to believe the first breastfeed will be blissful, think again. Your delicate nipple will be dragged far down the baby's palate and assaulted by hard little gums. It's not uncommon to muffle a yelping moan or instinctively want to push the mouth away. No one can really prepare you for the surprise but it proves there is good reason to roughly squeeze and pinch your nipples through pregnancy to toughen them up. By taking this approach there is a higher chance of avoiding nipple cracking later.

Fatigue is usually the most prevalent feeling with the first feed and you may not notice how efficient the child actually is in attaching easily. Nursing staff are happy even if there is only a small token feed before taking the baby off the breasts while they attend to ward preparation. The first feed is the beginning of a deep and abiding bonding process.

Bonding

There are many reports of women feeling an instant, incredible connection with their newborn baby, but what about the women who are not overwhelmed with blissful love responses? There are many women who do not feel this instant connection. Silent guilt for this apparent failing can consume their mind, wondering what is wrong with them. Admitting this lack of immediate love feels shameful so they keep their true feelings and reactions to themselves.

A lack of bond does not always mean the woman will turn her back on her baby. She might still cuddle, hold, feed and care for it with all her lovingness and attack anyone posing to cause harm. Yet within she is waiting for that 'ah ha' moment when she knows a deep and abiding love has arisen and oozes from the pores of her skin to the child. Perhaps the emotion of bonding and how it affects each person is different and comparisons only exist to cause emotional and mental strife.

Immediate bonding is obviously a beautiful experience for so many people. It is important to note, there is nothing wrong with a slower, delayed bonding while you process other parts of your emotional self. Caring for the child with gentleness and love, catering to all its immediate survival functions is enough.

Allow those feelings to unfold in your own time.

Bonding issues

Non-bonding can often be present when a mother has lost a child prior to this pregnancy and grieving has not completed itself. Often there are guilt feelings associated for loving the new baby when the baby who died no longer has a mother or a life. Feelings of betraying the love and memory of the child that did not live can become emotionally consuming, making bonding more difficult. It could lead into post-natal depression if not attended to.

Traumatic births can directly impact the ability to bond for both the mother and the father. Men who have to watch, powerless to help the labor and witness great damage to their partner might have retracted feelings and find it hard to open up to the baby. Even with an easy birth, sheer exhaustion might delay those feelings that other women feel immediately.

How a child was conceived could affect a mother's ability to reach out and open up. Accepting the baby into her life could mean she is forced to accept the events that led up to conception and her mind cannot allow her guard to fall down.

If any of these issues are still evident months into parenting, professional support is advised to help you process your reactions, delve into the causes and find some inner peace.

My Story

First Son

After the birth of my first son, the midwife laid his screaming little body on my chest. From my view, I saw an angry little waxy face screaming at me. My brain was still in birth mode, as though my consciousness was not fully present in the moment. I knew he was there yet all I could do was pat him. The birth had only been four hours and went like clockwork, so it's was not like I was overly fatigued or traumatized in any way, yet still I felt disconnected. Slowly patting him, I tried to take note of my surroundings, yet all the while my body began uncontrollably shaking. I did not pick up my son and cuddle or croon or say the words 'I love you'. Eventually the midwife told me to breastfeed and she picked him up and attached him to my nipple. That task completed, he was handed to my husband while a doctor prepared to stitch me up. So legs in the air, my mind is still out of it, the doctor proceeds to do his stitching work. Perhaps the pain began to anchor me in the present moment so when my boy was handed to me again, this time I cradled him close to me.

Now I do not really think this reaction is that strange. I became more worried when, arriving back in the ward, I defied every motherly instinct to remain close to my baby and never leave his side. Instead I left the poor little baby all by himself in the corner of the room by my bed and took off to the other side of the hospital, joining my husband to make phone calls. For me, I later judged myself for those actions as they went against all my thoughts of protecting the baby and having my energy and heart beat as close to him as possible to help him slowly adapt to the new environment. I had really strong ideas but did the opposite. I did, however, note when a nurse tried to take him from me later in the evening, I felt like a feral animal, wanting to grab my baby out of her clutching hands. The bonding was beginning. Two months later I felt myself suddenly fall in total love with my little boy.

Second Son

A great three-hour labor, my second son catapulted out and arrived into the world with speed. Full of fatigue, again I looked at my baby in a disconnected fashion; however, this time I managed to hold him, acting as I should act without a flushing of all those love chemicals rushing through me. Over the days and weeks that followed I eventually fell deeply in love with him.

This lack of instant bonding did not impact in any way my ability to nurture and care for my child. So if there are other ladies who feel similar to this, rest assured your development as a mother is unfolding in the correct time for you and the baby—comparisons will only make depression take hold, so remove that pressure.

Shaky Recovery

"Am I ok? My whole body feels like it is going into shock and I am shaking all over."

While all this confusion over feeding is taking place your body may start to shake uncontrollably. Not always apparent to the naked eye, the whole body may feel as though every atom, molecule and muscle is jittering, going through a massive release.

No one seems to notice your shaking or bewilderment because the midwives are either so used to it occurring they forget to tell you, or they are too busy cleaning up. Your partner will be so enmeshed in his own ecstatic fatherly reactions that he may not notice your distress. Rest assured the shaking is a normal part of the birth process.

It stands to reason that adrenaline, the fight/flight hormone, has been activated during labor and has now been released. Additional birth hormones are changing at this time. Besides, your body energy expenditure is as though you have just run a marathon, so of course when you stop suddenly, you will feel like collapsing in a shaking mess.

These shakes will subside after about ten minutes, just in time for the body to be taken over by another series of contractions, the placental birth. While waiting for this to occur, a series of medical checks are taking place.

Needles and Medical Check up

Labor and medical intervention is not over yet.

With baby wrapped up you might think you can settle into having quiet time without intervention. This will not be the case unless prior to going anywhere near a delivery suite you have made sure you know about all the injections and medical tests your baby will be put through directly after birth. Some of these tests you may not agree with and might choose to deny approval. This is up to you as you are now the legal guardian of the child and have the final say unless there are governmental laws in place saying otherwise. It's really important that all decisions are fully informed, and I suggest you seek out information about any side effects. Do your own research! If you decide to go ahead with all injections and medical intervention, know that some of those tests can be delayed for a while so you can ensure a total loving bond, before introducing pain to your little baby.

Medical staff are very business-like and do not have the time to explain every procedure they are doing. Often they will begin tests and give injections without really alerting you, assuming by your silence you have given permission.

Unfortunately stories are far too common of medical staff not informing or explaining medical procedures to the parents, thus not enabling them to give appropriate consent. You would think with new health and safety and insurance standard procedures in hospitals that medical staff should have already ensured that written consents have been gathered before labor even eventuated. This is often not the case and making fast rational decisions is extremely hard. I merely mention this due to the comments men and women have made in relation to their shock over injections and medical interventions that did not have to be made yet. Medical establishments may push their own agendas for ease of operation. For example, caesareans have radically increased and with these decisions so too has the emotional impact felt throughout families, as often depression can follow these choices.

*When exhausted from birthing you may not be feeling of **right mind** to make any decisions or to speak up and question staff on the day. Mistakes happen, so make sure your partner or support person is keeping an eye on proceedings and question on your behalf.*

Mother Gets an Injection

As you are giving birth, nursing staff will try to give you an injection in the thigh with an oxytocic agent, a drug that mimics the oxytocin effect to help the uterus contract after childbirth, assist the placental birth and avoid hemorrhaging. This sounds good, but is it really necessary? I requested waiting 15 minutes before an injection to see if my body could complete the process on its own. Close to 15 minutes the placenta cleared. Sometimes the micromanagement of birth and after care, in my opinion, interferes with natural processes. This is backed up by the ideas of Sarah Buckly MD, who offers an in-depth article with medical precision on this matter.

What to Expect

The Agpar Test – This is done twice in 5 minutes. Heart rate, breathing, activity and muscle tone, and skin color are all accessed to ensure your baby is healthy.

Vitamin K Shot – It's recommended in many Western countries to give a Vitamin K shot to assist with blood clotting. Newborn babies with low Vitamin K are at risk of dangerous bleeding.

Heel Pricks – These initially hurt the baby as they will squeal in pain. The heal prick is sent away for a multitude of tests to determine if your baby has any diseases. Liver function tests for jaundice are also detected via the heel prick.

Eye Care – Drops or ointment may be placed into the eyes when they first open them to minimize the transfer risk of STIs (sexually transmitted infections). Gonorrhea and Chlamydia infections can cause blindness in babies.

Hepatitis B Vaccine – Hepatitis B can cause lifelong infection, liver damage, and in some cases death. Generations ago, this vaccine was never given to newborn babies; nowadays it's given as a three-injection program. The first injection is given to your brand new baby at birth, followed by one in two months and another one suggested no later than 18 months.

Complete Check Up – measuring length, weight, height, temperature, and the staff will also attend to the umbilical cord. Sometimes they will wash the baby, other times they will advise refraining from washing for a few days.

Birth of the Placenta – Stage Three Labor

Contractions will rise and fall quite quickly, with a last sudden push to birth the placenta. This will rush out in a slithery mess full of more blood and slimy material. Nursing staff will studiously examine the placenta before disposing of it. They need to know that all components of the placenta has left your body; if any remains inside there is danger that you could end up with toxemia—essentially blood poisoning and infection. When the midwives are satisfied, they will prepare for a full clean up and await a doctor's appraisal on decisions around stitching.

Stitching – Birthing Stirrups

If an episiotomy (surgical cut) was performed or you tear while giving birth, surgical stitching will be required. Expect your legs to be unceremoniously placed apart, high in the air on a metal contraption, fondly called "birthing stirrups". This will have your vagina clearly visible to the doctor to give him the greatest visual ease and access to repair torn parts. Even with some local anesthetic this is not a pleasant experience.

As a mother who just gave birth, this is the last thing you want to be forced to deal with. There is no turning back; sadly, you must go through with it. You may not appreciate such intervention at the time; however, later you will be thankful for their expertise.

Return to the ward

Finally after all the stitching you will be instructed to go to the toilet and try to urinate. Nursing staff will want to hear of your success. Sometimes the body goes into so much shock that it cannot pass water; this could pose problems down the track. Padded up with maternity napkins you will be assisted back to the ward.

Monitoring and recording bowel and urine motions will be a routine part of your days while in hospital.

{ 4 }

Physical Recovery

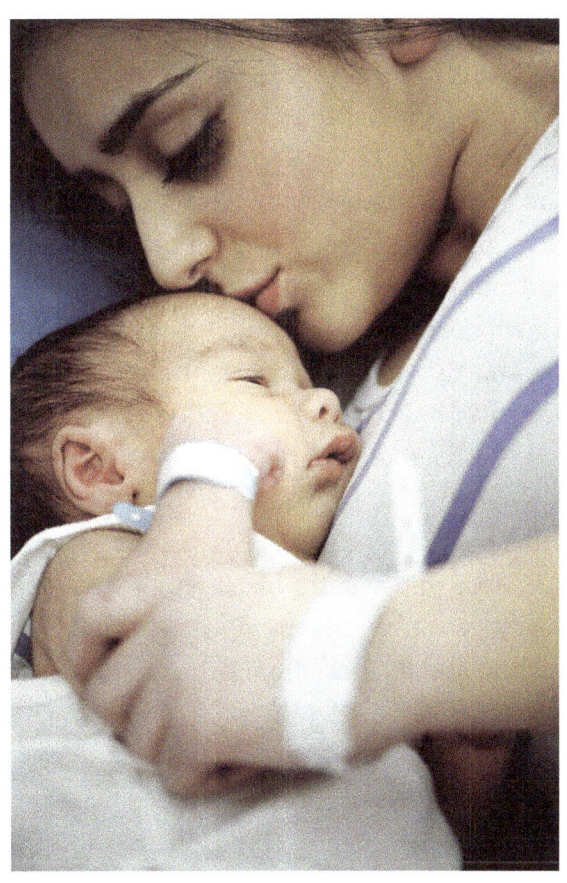

When Does Bleeding Stop and Sex Start?

"My husband is keen to begin making love straight away. When can we safely do this?"

Bleeding

Bleeding lasts for about two weeks but can go on for a month. The first week is like a heavier period with occasional gushing, often when breastfeeding. Small clots will also come away. The second week is similar to a normal period. Be aware, however, that if you start passing large clots in hospital then you must alert an on-duty nurse and if possible, show them the clots. That's right, as gruesome as it is you will have to fetch it from the toilet bowl or drag them in to see. I know you just want to die inside after reading this. I can assure you it is very important and the nurses will be avidly and medically interested in the clots if this is happening. These clots might be the result of placental residue that should have passed from the body at the time of birth. This could be an indication that the entire placenta did not detach from the uterus, now leaving you in potential danger of infection. Medical staff must be alerted. If infection occurs, blood poisoning can follow. Infections are not a good scenario.

I have encountered a few women who bled constantly for six weeks after the birth. This is not a usual occurrence and should be investigated. More importantly, bleeding for that long can cause iron deficiency, resulting in extreme fatigue and depression, so supplementation and medical monitoring is advised.

Sex

A six-week repair period is recommended before sexual intercourse. Bruising needs to ease, the vagina has to repair and the uterus is still retracting back into the original position prior to this time. Many women cannot contemplate sex for a long time after this. So if the pressure is on from your partner, do yourself a favor and just grab his appendage by the hand or be even more imaginative. The stress on him has been huge and often understated. Your man will thank you for it and it will give you hopefully another week to focus on the routine of parenting and internal body repair. The partner will feel loved and reassured that his needs will be met even though a baby is now taking up your life.

Medical Checks – Retracting Uterus and Bowel Movements

While in hospital, prepare to be subjected to many physical inspections of your post-baby body. Just when you thought all the poking would stop, there is more. Nursing staff will probe deeply into your abdomen to take specific uterus measurements. These measurements confirm if the uterus is retracting back to pre-conception size. All of this will be included in their medical notes, awaiting a doctor's perusal. Get ready for this delightful visit as he/she will need to inspect your lower regions. So before you know what is happening, you'll again have a head between your legs inspecting how your healing is progressing.

This may seem mortifying, however, it might help to be reminded how fortunate we are in the Western world to have such great medical care. Our sisters in third-world countries rarely have access to any qualified medical personnel, hygiene knowledge or after care.

As mentioned before, bowel movements become a subject of interest to the nursing staff. They need to know if your bowels are working properly before they discharge you from the hospital.

Tearing, Repair – Itchy Stitches

Being battered and bruised down below can make it difficult to sit upright. Stitches can add a new level of discomfort. Some ladies need a special cushion with a hole in it to lessen the pressure on the bruised areas or location of hemorrhoids. Sitting and walking adjustments are constantly required to alleviate tenderness. Trying to maintain a happy welcoming face to visitors while in recovery becomes an ordeal in itself.

By day three, stitches can dry out and become insanely itchy. It's hard to keep conversations going when all you want to do is scratch and tear at your vagina, seeking some form of relief. When walking, they pull and tug in different directions. At times they can tear and pull apart, requiring another stitch job. The good news is all these sensations are healthy signs of healing.

Soothing Sitz Baths and Ice – A sitz bath consists of warm water and a lot of salt. The salt aids in repair of the vaginal regions and soothes the discomfort of stitches. An ice pack is fantastic for a swollen uncomfortable vagina or hemorrhoids. Let an ice pack become your friend. The maternity ward will usually have some on hand. Make sure you speak up, as staff are not mind readers.

Floppy Baby Belly

"I still look pregnant!"

Added to your physical discomfort with your body under repair is the shocking realization that you still look fat even after the baby is born. The abdomen is still swollen like a beach ball, yet it is no longer tight and taut, it jiggles! What is that about? Forget the fantasy of jumping into pre-pregnancy clothing or looking fabulous for visitors. That all has to go on hold while you process this new body shape you are left with. Don't fear, most of the wiggly mass will go away after about two weeks, along with an average 5 kilos of weight loss. All that swelling is left over fluid from the pregnancy. Extra weight accrued after the initial loss will gradually disperse for most people when breastfeeding.

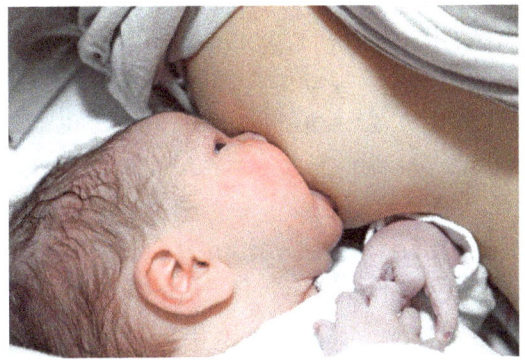

Breastfeeding Clumsiness

"I am useless, I cannot get the baby to attach!"

Who said breastfeeding is easy? It's the most ridiculous experience. Juggling the baby, trying every position, fumbling around, sucking, biting, change positions again. Breastfeeding is like a bloody circus act! I cannot explain it more bluntly than that. The whole experience in the first few days is fraught with tears, confusion, ineptness, fear of judgment and lack of coordination.

This expose is not going to be about how to correctly feed as there is no exact correct way, as every woman's nipple anatomy is different and the baby's capacity has a large part to play. Once you get over the initial shock of breastfeeding discomfort, you might have to go through the process of teaching the baby to do it properly. It's never explained to you that some babies have to actually be taught how to suck properly; it's not always a natural ability. Individual feeding abilities of the child can depend on the shape of nipples, how the mother holds herself, milk engorgement or unusually formed mouth palettes of the child.

Men hover around, anxious and perplexed as to why their partner does not seem to be able to manage breastfeeding when they are led to believe it is easy and the most natural pathway to be taken. Feeling inept to help or rectify the problem, he watches nervously, observing tears, anger, rejection of the baby, tantrums and retries all within an hour. Then it starts again on the next feed. The woman usually feels a failure, floundering hopelessly with the inability to become comfortable and at ease with feeding. This whole experience is worsened due to her need to know she can ensure her baby's survival and to also prove her female prowess to her partner and others in this department.

The whole process is completely frustrating and takes time to become comfortable and efficient. Banana pillows can be really useful to help bolster the elbow and arm as you try to position the baby into the best feeding position. Nurses will do whatever they can to help you within their time constraints; be aware, however, of the very brisk nurse that becomes impatient when asking for help. Facing an impatient nurse in this delicate stage of mothering can cause undue scarring on your confidence. Many women, myself included, have faced one of these highly efficient women who huff and puff over to you, snatch the baby from your arms, bundle them up and then thrust their little mouths over your nipple, all the while, without warning, squeezing, pinching the nipple flat, shoving it towards the open hungry mouth. Not only do you feel humiliated by this onslaught, you actually feel assaulted. This is most unfortunate for a new mother as behavior like this is enough to create resistance of asking for help, leaving her in a predicament. Her continued confidence before leaving hospital relies on this early training.

Professional trained lactation consultants are available for separate training and support. This might be recommended when:
- A woman has flat or inverted nipples. The baby's mouth finds it hard to attach.
- Cleft palette babies sometimes can have major problems with feeding if parts of the upper palette are missing; suction becomes difficult.
- Tongue tie can adversely affect the depth of the latch on for sufficient connection.
- Elongated time in a neo natal crib, fed by a line. There is potential for the baby to forget the sucking action as the milk is drip fed with a line directly into the stomach via the nose so the baby forgets how to suck and attach properly.

My Story

Lazy drinking due to jaundice

First son was an extremely tired baby, barely able to stay attached for long on the breast and was beginning to lose weight. I tried hard to keep him feeding but he would go floppy and fall off. Eventually a nurse finally took notice and realized he had become quite jaundiced, resulting in his liver having to work too hard to remove and replace blood cells. They had to place him in a neo natal crib under lights. Luckily I was able to take him out for short spurts to feed him and noticed his strength increased. We discovered his body was battling my blood that had flushed back through the placenta at the time of birth and his little body was trying to clear it.

Memory loss due to elongated neo natal care

My second son was born and within one day he began turning yellow, so the doctor was alerted. A heel prick confirmed he had severe jaundice for the same reason as my first son. He was taken and placed under lights for five consecutive days and was not allowed out for feeding. He was drip fed a line and when he eventually came out he had no idea how to feed. He screamed and roared at me as his hungry mouth hunted for the food. He could smell it but did not realize he had to attach and suck.

We had to see a lactation consultant and visit her daily while my son was given mouth physiotherapy exercises to teach him to open his mouth wide. In the meantime I expressed and fed him with a line attached to my finger. Eventually as he learnt to open his mouth I could attach the line to my nipple so when he attached he would get instant gratification and introduce the mouth sucking action. Finally we were able to successfully remove the line and have him feed properly. It was an epic journey lasting two weeks. The whole process of expressing, feeding and sleeping before the next meal took nearly two hours. My babies fed every two and half hours as both babies seemed to have small stomach capacity or my milk production was on the low side. So half hour sleeps between feeds took its toll; however, we pushed through and it was worth it.

Breastfeeding and attachment only gets harder when the milk comes in and the breasts become engorged.

Engorgement – The Milk Comes

"I am dying inside every time I feed my baby, the pain is excruciating."

"When I feed my baby I suffer intense pain in the uterus just like when I was in labor."

After Pains

Often with second babies but rarely with the first, women can experience contractions when breastfeeding, known as 'after pains'. These contractions can be as severe as labor contractions. The intensity can take your breath away, making it difficult to stay focused on nursing.

It's quite common when back in the ward for the nursing staff to walk around giving out painkillers. With my first child I was mystified as to why all the women were accepting pain killers. I had to phone my mother to ask her, as I didn't want to appear ignorant. She explained how feeding your baby activates the contractions to help the uterus shrink back to normal size. With this information now locked away, I decided to watch the faces of my neighbors, and sure enough they were certainly in a level of pain that I wasn't feeling. My second baby gave me first-hand experience of this.

For the first three days the baby is drinking colostrum known as the 'fore milk'; this is filled with antibodies used for building their immune systems. It is usually after day three that the proper milk comes in.

Medical staff may come and ask if your milk has come in. New mothers will assume that the milk has come in because the baby is drinking. If unsure about the milk coming in at this point, there will be absolutely no doubt when it does. The breasts become engorged and so full of milk that it'll feel like you've had the worst kind of breast implants. Engorgement is an understatement to the condition that really happens.

The breasts become full and painfully swollen, heavy and rock solid to the touch. They will feel like two rocks that you could rip off your chest and throw away as far as they will go. They leak everywhere and leave sticky wet patches over your clothes and sheets. Not only is the breast enlarged but the nipple swells in epic proportions and the once delicate button-like nipple resembles nothing you have seen before. If the nipple shape has drastically changed, making it extremely difficult for the baby to wrap their mouth around it, frustration will follow. The tug of war between frustrated baby and mother begins. If your nipples are already cracked at this time, then tears of pain are common at each feeding. I have seen women sob with pain while still trying to nourish their child.

If they were not cracked before engorgement then they usually become cracked afterwards. This is due to the child's ferocious gums munching down on engorged nipple tissue while trying to get the whole nipple into the mouth.

Client Story

"After the birth, my breasts continued to increase in size until both of them were huge shiny conical shapes. The pain and pressure inside them felt intense. Milk spurted over my clothes and upon the floor. I felt like I could feed an office block. Medical staff requested photographs and video footage for training purposes, as they had never seen a case as severe as mine. To complicate the matter, I was told if I expressed the milk from my distorted nipples to help my baby attach, I could inadvertently cause greater milk production."

Managing Engorgement

When breasts fill up to the degree that the baby cannot drink properly, midwives and nurses suggest that you should express some of the milk first before trying to feed. "How do you do that?" one might ask. Vague comments from rushed nurses just say "Get in the shower and massage the area and allow the milk to drip out." Another comment might be to push down the breast in an action towards the nipple and milk will miraculously flow out. *Well sadly, it is not always as easy as that.*

If you can't express properly, midwife attention may be required. Look out! They can be aggressive, matter of fact and hurried! They grab your painful nipples and forcefully squeeze the breasts and nipple. If you are seeking their help for breastfeeding, they again squeeze the breast and nipple then shove your baby's mouth over the top and push the baby's head against your chest. The process is so quick there is barely any time to yelp. If you have never felt emotionally or mentally abused before, you will after. For a new mother, a midwife's practical, intense approach can be overwhelmingly frightening. For me, one midwife was lucky she didn't get a smack across her head. Actually, I was too frightened she'd smack me back!

To give them credit, they are overworked and new mothers are high maintenance. They know their job and although their attitude may be dauntingly brisk they get the desired results. So, despite the frustration you as a new mother may go through, you just have to keep persevering with the methods they show.

Prior to a feed, midwives may help by suggesting you have a warm shower. The warm shower allows the milk to flow and ease the pressure on the breast from the excess milk. You will usually need to massage or strip the breast to increase the amount of milk loss. Do this by moving your thumb down towards the nipple in deep stroking actions, making sure the pressure is consistent. The rest of your hand should be underneath the breast to support it. As the thumb nears the nipple, squeeze and push with the fingers underneath the breast and the thumb at the top, pushing towards the nipple. Hopefully some milk will come out, but not always. It is painful to squeeze and stroke the breast while it is engorged so a new mum will often hesitate to use the pressure required to rid the breast of the excess milk.

This is a difficult process to explain in writing. It sounds easy but it is not when it's your first time. To have someone demonstrate with their breast would visually help. Trying to find someone who will do this for you could be quite difficult. You could always ask your mother. Physical demonstrations speak louder than words.

Here is a helpful video link http://www.nhs.uk/conditions/pregnancy-and-baby/pages/expressing-storing-breast-milk.aspx#close

Cold Cabbage Leaves

Placing cold cabbage leaves inside your bra can ease severe cases of engorgement. This will give some relief but should not be used frequently as the cabbage leaf's action will dry up the milk. Cabbage leaves aid milk absorption back into the body away from the breasts. Most maternity wards have cabbage leaves in their refrigerators for patients who need to completely dry up their milk. Listen to staff as they will advise if this is appropriate for your situation. The humble cabbage leaf has reportedly been used since the 1800s It is theorized that inherent qualities in the cabbage improves blood flow in and out of the area, assisting trapped fluid in the breast. For more interesting information see this link: http://www.lactationconsultant.info/cabbagecure.html

Machines for Expressing

You have probably organized or thought about a small hand pump in case you need to express milk at any time. Handheld pumps are difficult to use, mainly because first time users find everything about breasts and milk awkward. It's easy to become frustrated, possibly even embarrassed. But you'll be relieved to know the process becomes easier with time and practice, so persevere past the give up point, knowing that with engorgement comes pain until the pressure is released. Unfortunately, giving up results in more discomfort due to the continuous production of milk. If at all possible get your hands on an electric machine pump; they are blissful and easy to use, even if you feel like a cow in a dairy shed. Hospitals usually have some available to use during your stay. Long-term use can be arranged through a rental company that deals in these devices. Sometimes lactation clinics have them for hire.

If all else fails and you cannot possibly persist with breastfeeding, your next choice is the bottle.

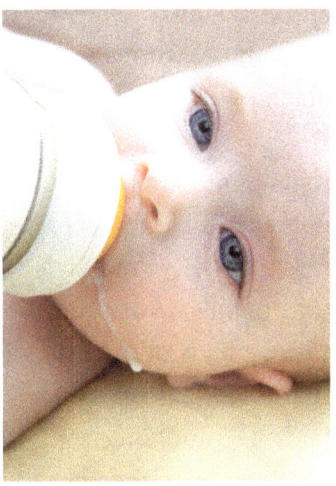

Bottle Feeding

"I can't wean my child, she just won't go to the bottle."

"My baby hates the bottle, he'll drink for a while but then starts screaming as though he is angry."

The type of milk formula to use should be chosen at the parents' investigation and discretion. It is not my role to suggest one type of formula over another. My interest in bottle-feeding has more to do with how you can successfully convert your child from the breast to the bottle in the least problematic way.

Changing from breast to bottle could be for a variety of personal reasons. In this modern age, Western mothers are required to return to work early just to make ends meet. Some mothers rejoin the workforce as a way of regaining some sanity or to pay the bills; other mothers may not have enough breast milk and will need to supplement feeds. Regardless of the reason for needing to bottle feed, the changeover process can be fraught with difficulties. The most common is the emotional guilt and sadness that both mother and child are missing out on essential emotional bonding. Secondly, changing from a soft nipple to a hard rubbery one can be quite challenging for the baby to understand how to effectively feed.

A baby knows that a bottle nipple is not the same as the breast. This is understandable as the baby experiences breastfeeding as a holistic sensory process where they feel the soft flesh upon the cheek and the sound of the heart pounding in their ears while sucking the nipple to the back of its throat and tugging on it with gusto. Breastfeeding for mothers can be a comforting experience once routine is established and once the nipples are not so sensitive. Baby and mother can relax together in a beautiful way.

Imagine what it is like for the baby, who has experienced that wonderful sensory process only to be presented with a hard, cold nipple of a bottle that doesn't go to the back of the throat, and pressed up against harsh knitwear or clothes that rub against their soft cheek. Added to that, the clear pounding of the mother's heart is replaced with a muffled version because of clothes interfering with the clarity of sound sensations. The baby now has some good reasons to be suspicious of the bottle-feeding method.

Gradual Change Over

Get rid of your top when trying to introduce the bottle. Allow your baby the security of introducing one change to its normal feeding sensations at a time. The child will adapt far better to the hard nipple if all other known senses are present. This process will also be comforting for the mother as a sense of bonding can still be experienced.

Over time you can slowly eliminate the sensation of skin on skin and the dependence on the mother's heartbeat. Men also can feed their babies this way and allow a fatherly bonding. A baby in utero can hear sounds of the outside world and to a lesser degree will be aware of the father's heart beat signals.

A natural bare-breasted approach is especially vital for any woman who finds that she cannot breastfeed at all. If a woman finds herself in this position, deep emotional distress, guilt and feelings of feminine inadequacy are usually present. This approach allows women and their babies to experience the same bonding sensations minus the real nipple. This process can bridge the psychological gap and offer healing moments to the distressed mother.

Relationship Bonding

I believe early bottle-feeding with expressed milk is a must for both parents to do. When a baby enters the household, so too does chaos. The level of involvement required to care for a child is quite daunting. Outings with a wife or a partner now come with a helpless bundle of arms and legs, full of demands and needs. This new set of circumstances can be quite a shock to both mother and father. Mothers often become depressed if their normal active lifestyle is suddenly squashed, so it stands to reason that a balanced approach needs to be found to reduce confusion and prevent resentment from arising.

If you can introduce early versatility to the feeding methods, some of these pressures can be alleviated. Mothers can find a moment of peace by going for a walk while the father bonds through feeding their child. Grandparents can feel needed and will also be able to form early relationships with their grandchildren. Fathers will be relieved to find some normalcy to their life if they can have some exclusive time with their partner.

Protective instincts of a mother are often too strong in the first three months to extract her from the baby and allow for these outings to occur. It takes time before her protectiveness allows other people to be more helpful and supportive. Patience is a huge factor at this time.

Over Tight Bottle Lid

Babies being introduced to a bottle early may seem to be keen on sucking but then throw their heads back as though they are angry that a bottle and not a breast have been given to them. Other babies may suck for their life and get so tired that they fall asleep without drinking much at all. If this happens, pay attention to the bottle lid. When you first feed the baby you may notice a trickle of bubbles going from the bottom of the bottle to the top. This trickle of bubbles indicates that milk is moving out of the nipple opening. If the bubbles stop it means the child has either stopped sucking or a vacuum has developed and no matter how hard the baby sucks it can't get any more milk. No new air is coming into the bottle to allow the flow of milk.

If this happens and milk flow is nonexistent there is a good chance the baby will become frustrated with the lack of milk forthcoming. They show this by throwing their heads around screaming blue murder. Babies who have exhausted themselves with frantic sucking will eventually just give up and go to sleep. When they next wake (earlier than a usual feed) they will be starving, resulting in another bout of screaming, especially if another bottle is given that again does not provide adequate milk flow. I have seen this happening time and time again with mothers who present at my clinic or seek advice over the phone.

Adjusting the bottle: If you tighten the bottle lid too much you will reduce the airflow in the bottle and once the baby sucks, a vacuum effect will form. When tightening the lid you should turn it until you can't turn anymore and then half turn the other way. Place the bottle in the baby's mouth and see if a continuous flow of bubbles and a slight whistling can be seen and heard. If the bubbles are present the lid is allowing enough air in to continue with successful feeding. If the bubbles start but quickly stop again take the bottle from the baby's mouth and loosen it a little more or until you notice the bubbles rising to the surface. Once you see a thread of bubbles continuing up to the surface you have reached the right level. If you cannot see the line you may hear a small trailing bubble sound.

Cracked Nipples

"I can't do it anymore, feeding is so painful."

"It should not be this hard."

Until you experience it, you can't imagine the searing, shooting pain that occurs as a result of cracked nipples. Tiny cracks might give rise to some pain but it's far worse when the nipples are really cracked and almost bloody. The daily onslaught of a baby's munching gums through breastfeeding, shows no mercy, when the milk comes in, the nipples become distorted and enlarged making it even more difficult for the baby to find best mouth placement for sucking. A baby does not consider your pain it's only focused on survival. Breastfeeding with cracked nipples becomes a groaning, agony filled nightmare. Proper nipple care at this stage is a must, with possible expressing for a while to allow recovery. Cracked nipples can lead to mastitis, a milk duct infection that causes sharp pain within the breast tissue. Progressive mastitis will cause body health to decline.

Nipple management

Express for a while to allow your nipples to repair and seek extra medical support in case your breastfeeding style or nipple formation encourages the baby to latch on and feed incorrectly. Do not put creams on the nipples as it softens them even more. Sunlight is a fantastic healer, so any chance you have, reveal your breasts to the sun. Lavender oil, as mentioned earlier, can be placed around the breast to avoid infections—make sure you use it away from feeding times. If you must use a cream it should be zinc based, as zinc is known for its great skin healing properties.

Day Three: Emotional Uproar

"I can't stop crying."

By day three your milk will be fully coming in, and with it comes a change in releasing hormones that could send you into a freaky, crying mess. Both you and your partner could become confused and not understand why the high of birth has suddenly dropped, or why angry words are spoken. There is no need for alarm; it's normal and after a day or two it will pass. Help your partner know it's not really him, even though you may have blurted otherwise. It's just another phase you have to pass through.

Many women have found that evening primrose oil supplements can help regulate the hormone release and lessen the worst of those emotional outbursts without harming the baby. Regardless of possible supplement support you will move through this phase.

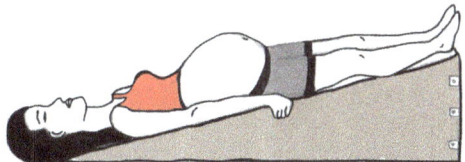

Lack of Uterus Strength – Pelvic Floor Muscles

"I feel like my uterus is going to drop out at any moment."

Having a baby is a huge ordeal for the body. Pelvic floor muscles have been stretched beyond normal function and take a while to spring back with strength and vitality. When walking around after having a baby, **some women** comment on feeling like their uterus is going to drop out. Sneezing, running, coughing, or jumping can make that sensation seem worse. Cautious walking, contracting and pulling all your muscles up towards the head emphasizes this feeling. For many women this disconcerting feeling might only last for a couple of weeks, especially with a first child; however, it has been known to last up to six months on rare occasions.

Quick movements, running or jumping may not be something eagerly pursued. This condition might also create a fear of sex, thinking penile insertion might loosen internal muscles. Pelvic floor muscle exercises are paramount to helping the body make a full recovery, but time and patience are also essential. Hospital physiotherapists can assist with providing specific exercises. Some hospitals have a physiotherapist come to the ward and speak with each new mother and may even organize a group instruction session.

Prolapse of the Uterus

In extreme cases through birth, the uterus may prolapse. Through difficult births, large babies or prolonged pushing, pelvic floor muscles can weaken or even become damaged. There are four stages to a prolapse. Stage one is where the uterus protrudes into the upper part of the vagina. In stage two, the uterus has descended almost to the opening of the vagina. Stage three reveals the uterus protruding out of the vagina and in extreme cases stage four is when the uterus is completely distended out of the vagina. In a worst case scenario surgery may be required; in less serious situations surgical rings may be placed inside the vagina to help reinforce the walls until the muscles strengthen.

In most cases, especially first births, there is a greater likelihood of slight weakening or stage one prolapse. In this situation daily pelvic floor exercises are effective and essential. Using a slant board and the force of gravity while doing the exercises will prove to be more effective and with quicker results, and will strengthen the pelvic muscles to a deeper degree. Sadly, caesarean births might not provide a safe haven from this situation. Sometimes the prolapse occurs even from carrying a large baby to full term.

What is a slant board? This is a board made in your home that lays with one part resting on the floor and the other on the side of the bed. You lie down fully on the board with feet facing towards the ceiling and head towards the ground. This creates a gravity effect, where the uterus and any other organs involved in the prolapse will slowly move back towards the abdominal region within the pelvic cavity. The board may have rope loops to hold your feet in place so you don't fall off. Once you are in this position you can begin your pelvic floor exercise routine. Alternatively, a local gymnasium will usually have an incline bench and this will serve the same purpose.

Incontinence

Urinary incontinence can be a common complaint after the birth. Downward pressure of the abdomen by sudden sneezing, coughing, or sudden movements can cause small amounts of urine to escape. This can be quite embarrassing as you sit or walk around worrying if other people can see the leakage. For some women leakage can be quite severe, causing great anxiety over the idea that they are stuck with this forever. New mothers may find it hard to admit this to anyone, as urination and bowel movements are a private affair. There is also pride and privacy that get in the way. However ,your doctor can provide a referral to a physiotherapist who will design special exercises to remedy the problem. Pilates is also a great therapy for strengthening your core muscles and usually involves some pelvic floor exercises.

In some cases, especially with third and fourth degree tears, a woman might end up with major incontinence, resulting in follow-up surgeries. Vaginal tearing of this degree could cause a variety of other internal issues along with emotional upheaval.

Washing and Dressing the Baby

"Everyone is staring at me, judging me."

"I cannot change my baby, I feel like I am going to break her."

Washing

One of the greatest joys a couple can have is bathing their child. There is something really beautiful about a baby submerged in the water, blissfully floating in the warmth and this provides a wonderful connection time. That joy only remains if your baby actually enjoys the bathing process. Every parent feels inept and concerned when dealing with a tiny, floppy-headed baby that becomes slippery with water. Under the watchful eye of a nurse, confidence will soon be ensured. Don't stress over washing daily as disrobing and clothing the baby tires them since they not used to being handled so much. Remember a newborn has just left a world filled with water and gentle caressing movements, not pull, tug and grab. Try not to let other people's opinions force you to over-wash the baby at this delicate stage. This is a great time for fathers to feel they can have a direct involvement in the care and nurturing of their baby and this connection time should be encouraged.

Difficulties in Dressing your Baby for the First Time

If you think holding, handling, breastfeeding and washing your baby is awkward, then wait until it's time to dress him or her. Their little arms and legs seem so breakable and when trying to poke their hands and legs through some of the fancy clothes you have bought it becomes really difficult to control. Women often nervously look around to see if anyone has noticed the clothing struggle, often feeling humiliated and judged because they appear uncoordinated and seemingly inept. This is another area where you think it should be second nature to dress your baby, yet when faced with the reality it is a completely different story. Every mother feels this way, so even if you share a ward with experienced women who have just had their second or third child, remember they too once felt the same with their first baby. No one is judging you, except yourself. Deeper anxiety might arise if you believe your partner is also judging your ability to mother correctly. Frayed tempers and crying are common emotional states associated with these thoughts and feelings.

To make this adjustment time easier it is best to choose clothes that require the least limb handling. As mentioned before, babies become tired and fractured by too much handling, so you are doing yourself and the newborn a favor by choosing sensible clothes that are easy to get on and off, rather than fancy cute ones to greet visitors with.

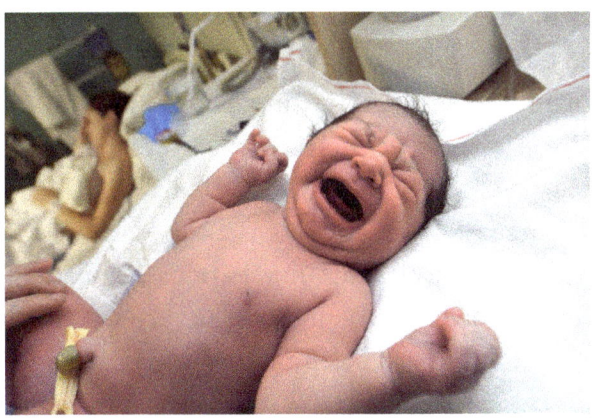

Umbilical Cord Care

We often mistakenly assume a newborn baby is born with a beautiful navel and perfect smooth abdomen. If you have not had much access to a naked newborn baby then you might not realize there is still some major healing the baby must do in order to adjust to this world. When finally coming out of the labor daze, seeing the baby's naked body for the first time might cause you some alarm. A baby's genitals are much larger than you would expect and can be swollen; but never fear, they will grow into them or swelling will subside. You'll also be faced with a navel that looks like it exploded. From the first visual surprise, on closer inspection you will see a part of the placenta hanging off the navel, red and swollen but crimped with a plastic clamp. Do not worry though, as the umbilical cord doesn't contain sensitive nerve fibers that relay pain, so the baby is quite comfortable. Your baby's navel will look like this for a few days, but over of the next two weeks the remaining placenta will dry and shrivel up and disconnect, leaving the baby, in most cases, with a perfectly normal looking navel.

Caring for the stump

The umbilical cord stump will change from yellowish green to brown and then black before falling off.

Minimizing downward pressure on the healing stump will ensure there is not early tearing before correct healing takes place so that the navel does not become infected.

Keep Clean and Dry – It's important to keep the stump clean and dry with access to clear air flow. In humid climates its best for the diaper to be rolled down under the navel and the baby should wear light cotton shirts so perspiration and overheating is kept to a minimum.

There are various thoughts around washing. Some medical practitioners suggest sponge bathing your child until the umbilical cord heals. If you are more inclined to enjoy the process of submerging your baby in water then it is important that drying is completed by holding a dry cloth around the stump.

Drying by sunlight can also be a great way to increase the healing.

Do not pull it off – Don't pull off the last remaining strands no matter how tempting it may be. Any forcible tearing could create an open wound, with possible infection as a result.

Newborn Black Tar Poo – Meconium

"My baby's poo is sticky and green. What is wrong with her?"

If you choose to wash the whole baby every few days then all you have to really attend to in between washes is their bottom. Early baby poo is not light brown like you may think. It's actually greeny-black and extremely sticky and hard to wipe off. Seeing the black poo for the first time can be a shock, especially when nursing staff forget to tell you this is normal. The black fecal matter is a residue of dead red blood cells that have been rapidly replaced once the baby is born and breathing on its own, no longer reliant on the mother. This usually happens around 24 hours after birth.

Two to four days after birth the poo changes. Poo can be green in color and less tacky in consistency. This is a great sign that your baby's intestinal tract is developing smoothly. From here on in, changes in baby poo color and consistency coincide with changes to food and health; soon you will receive nappies full of frothy explosive breastfeeding poo or firmer ones when bottle-feeding. They are little poo machines that never stop.

{ 5 }

A New Family Member

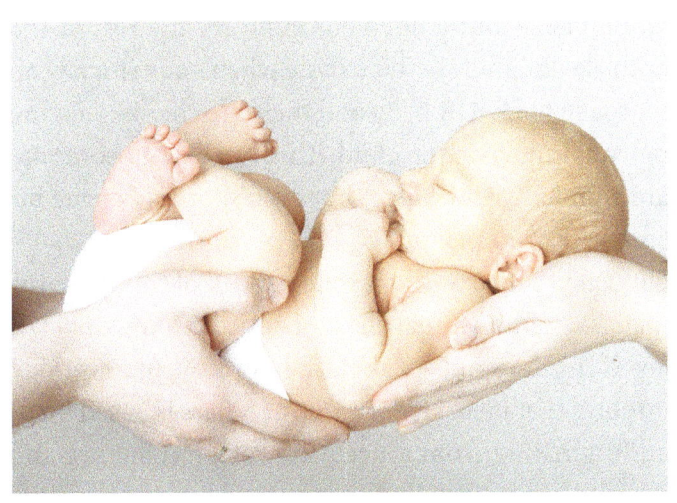

You are Now a Parent

Now a parent, your whole life perspective will change. Parenting heralds in new levels of responsibility, affecting you in ways that could never be imagined. Sole care for this little person who completely trusts you to keep him/her safe can cause unusual attitudes. Overprotective behaviors, control freak reactions, and adjusted expectations from partners all come together, morphing you into a person that you barely know and are having to get used to.

It's not uncommon for relationships with family members to become strained as you begin developing ideas on how you wish to raise, influence and guide your child for the rest of their life. Parents-in-law might lose their shine when you critically appraise their approach to YOUR baby and their life choices that might, in the long run, influence the child. This can lead to some stressful, awkward moments with them, but even more so, create hurt and confusion with your partner.

In clinical practice, I hear women speak of this issue time and time again. When a woman has a baby she immediately calls it *her* baby. If she does not speak it, she thinks it and every decision wraps around that idea. Her critique of others is based on her perception, originating from a need to protect, influence and grow her baby into a successfully functioning human being. She is so determined and adamant in relation to this, that partners can be placed on the back seat, and their opinions and personal needs to also have a say in child rearing are often overlooked or fought about. Many times those thoughts and opinions were never discussed or perceived until the birth of the child, thus surprising both parents and placing unusual strain on this constantly morphing relationship.

Give my Baby Back! Instinctual Protectiveness

"I don't want anyone touching my baby."

When visitors start to turn up do not be surprised if you have a huge reaction around people grabbing at your baby, picking it up or uncovering it, or worse still, waking it up with insistent requests for cuddling. Some mothers become completely overwhelmed with ferocious feelings of protectiveness and do not want anyone touching their baby. They can even have difficulty watching a partner clumsily hold onto it. Those feelings are not often spoken about because the mother feels a little ashamed and even shocked by her raw emotions and unexpected resistance. Her fear of being labeled unfriendly, neurotic, nasty or purposefully hurtful can silence her deepest feelings, yet she may still appear agitated.

Speaking up is difficult as friends will not understand and feel personally wounded, also judging such reactions as abnormal. Women and girls without children are sometimes desperate to get their hands on any baby so they can experience the maternal instinct. They may have no point of reference to your feelings so a little compassion might be easier to muster, but women who are parents themselves and have been through the process of birth should know better. When they behave in demanding ways it can be downright annoying. They will activate an anger response faster than anyone.

It is important to honor those feelings should they arise by requesting a little space and adjustment time. By two weeks those intense feelings will diminish once there is reassurance your baby is healthy and safe. In the end, it is your baby and not the property of all the visitors. These emotions and reactions are completely natural but not openly spoken of. You have given birth to a child that previously was encased in a germ-free, completely hygienic, sanitized space for nine months. It's up to you to protect them. Now they are in the world, unprotected, and reliant on your ability to protect them.

To ensure your baby's survival, their immune system must strengthen. In truth, early introduction to many people and their associated germs and bacteria could pose a threat to your baby's development. In general terms, as a society we don't worry too much about this and babies survive regardless. For many women this protective feeling is more a subconscious instinctual one, more in line with the animal kingdom. When we scrutinize our existence, there are many aspects of behavior that mimic animal behavior in the wild. So it's not unreasonable to suggest some women feel protective more than others, and will act in unusual ways to ensure no one touches their baby, until she feels a safe period of time has passed.

It would be remiss of me to forget to mention the situation of hurt feelings experienced when an excited mother encounters people who do not jump for joy to grab her child or gasp with delight over her new bundle. Not everyone will be immersed in your journey into parenthood and have their reason why they prefer to not hold your baby. You need to quietly respect their stance without acting rejected or on the attack. If you note hesitancy in their body language then don't thrust the baby at that person. Everyone has their own story as to why they act and feel the way they do. You also need to be mindful that many women suffer grief and loss through pregnancy and might not wish to confront those feelings. Some people just don't do babies.

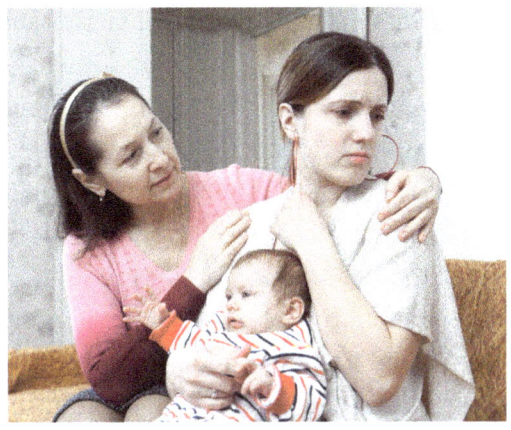

Mothers and Mothers-in-law
Anxiety and Resentment Begin

"It makes me angry when my mother-in-law tells me how to look after my baby."

The hardest people to deny holding the baby will be your mother or mother-in-law and female grandparents. These women sometimes act as though it's their divine right to have complete access to your baby. In some ways, early introduction ensures they create an energetic bond with your child that will keep developing as the child grows. As a young mum, *do not* underestimate the loving support available to you that could be called upon at a moment's notice with this tribe of older women. Bonding can be important and better timing for this to occur might need to be negotiated.

A new mother often feels threatened and judged by the aging women. Due to nervousness and self-doubt, she prefers her inability to be a supermom to remain unknown. A calm, collected exterior hides an anxiety-filled mind. In her view these female elders have already proven their success at parenting. Knowing this, the younger woman fears they are criticizing and judging her every move. Feelings of inadequacy and irritation is increased when comments that are offered with helpful intention are barked out like intrusive demands by pushy family members who think you should parent your child like they did.

Grandparents have often told me that when their daughter or daughter-in-law is not around, they purposefully feed the child food that is on the mother's taboo list. The grandmother has made her own judgments about what she believes is right for another woman's child and had totally ignored the parents' request. This behavior does not allow the open, trusting relationships of grandparents to grow in a positive way. Instead, it opens up a hurtful and damaging battlefield. Respect and acceptance is crucial for a new mother to feel she has earned her rightful place in society and family need to back off to let her discover her own version of parenting.

Please keep in mind as a new parent you are highly sensitive to everyone and everything in your environment. Perception of criticism and judgment might be tainted by self-doubt. Helpful, and sometimes overly helpful comments, based on love and support may actually be interpreted as criticism. Verbally lashing out could result in pushing your greatest supporters away. Tread carefully and develop language that values their input, but assert the need to discover this new path on your own, gently reminding them you are the parent, not them. Reassure them that requests for help and advice will be asked when the need arises. Your mother and mother-in-law want nothing more than your greatest success.

Having said that, I have heard accounts where mothers-in-law especially have stated direct ownership of the baby and state they will do whatever they like when looking after the baby. In some strange way they actually believe it is their property. If you are faced with this, please seek some counseling support to help you find ways to navigate this difficult problem.

Listening to Advice or Words of Encouragement

You may feel a natural resistance to listen to caring people's advice, unfortunately gems of wisdom could be missed that would make all the difference to your parenting confidence and baby comfort. I learnt to mostly listen to my mother and found her advice to be very sound and incredibly helpful. She did pass on great knowledge having birthed eight children. Her wisdom and common sense were really important to me. There were some instances where I thought I knew better, only to find myself eating humble pie and admit she was right. Learning to listen and respect her observations quickly replaced my youthful pride.

Each generation has its own vanity and sense of superiority when it comes to raising a child. A common view that older women's wisdom is outdated and irrelevant is on the rise, since we now have easy access to the internet and a plethora of attitudes and views. However, you will soon realize that nothing can replace the experience of a woman who has nurtured children of her own and is willing to support you. Sometimes it's actually worth listening, in case you learn something not shared or even considered important to share in our multimedia world.

Fear of Judgment

"I become really anxious when in groups or in public and people are looking at me."

"I feel like I cannot live up to my new mother role."

One of the most taxing experiences a new mother can go through is the constant negative self-talk of her own mind. Staying at home with your baby, hidden from the world, might help to avoid your worst insecurities, but they soon rage out of control once you step foot outside. Wherever you go it can feel like everyone is looking at you as though under a microscope. A new baby becomes a supersonic magnet attracting all manner of people who want to touch, poke or talk to it. You feel like everyone is watching and judging every move you make, deciding on your worthiness to be a mother. This extreme sense of focalized attention puts huge pressure on your shoulders and only reinforces the inner anxieties.

Public Breastfeeding

Most new mothers choose to remain at home when it's breastfeeding time as they often feel inept and awkward when first learning to successfully attach their baby to the nipple. There is also a skill to feeding in public and keeping yourself modest so as to not cause undue attention. New mothers take a while to eliminate awkward feeding postures. When they see other mothers so easily resuming the breastfeeding position it doesn't help their confidence.

If you choose to feed in public places, a modesty cloth is easy to carry. You can feed by placing the cloth or baby's blanket over your shoulder and then lift it up slightly while attaching your baby to the nipple. It is as easy and as simple as that. There is no real reason for showing a lot of flesh.

Pregnancy and Birth: The Conspiracy of Silence

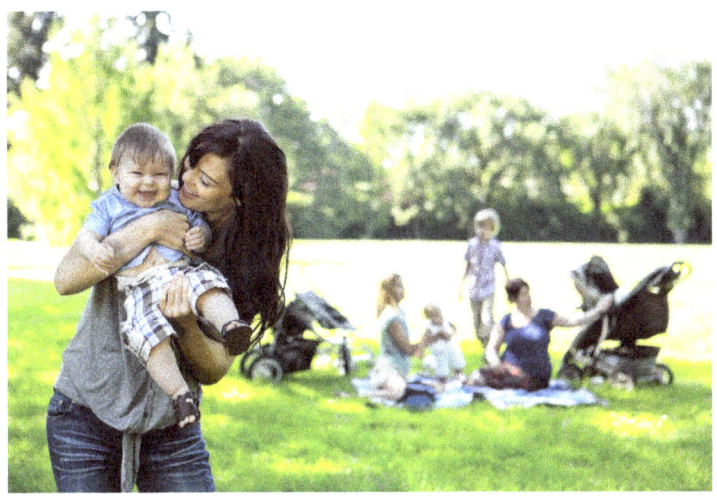

Mother's Groups

At least for the first few months, try to avoid mothers groups. I would say avoid them at all costs, or at least for a few months. Having heard so many distressing stories in my natural therapies and counseling clinic over the years, I am convinced these groups can do more harm than good. In many ways it helps to have other moms to speak to for reassurance, especially in relation to your baby's growth and development stages. This should be a positive opportunity, yet involvement in these groups often increases stress and anxiety.

Insecurities are already part of the parenting vocabulary. It does not serve to have any of them magnified by random, snippy comments from other women who look like they have their life and parenting under control. Mothers groups are a breeding ground for distress as they create their own weird little environment of competition, life comparisons and one-upmanship. Sometimes shared experiences are not the raw truth, leading the listener into a spiral of doubt. It must be remembered that women do not always tell the truth in fear they will be judged in a negative light.

My clinic is filled with the tears of women struggling because they went to these groups too early. Often they want to leave but don't know how to extract themselves from the group in fear of causing offence, especially if they have made lovely connections with some of the other mothers.

Breastfeeding Groups

If normal mothers groups are bad, the vigilante behavior of breastfeeding groups are worse. These women all profess a great desire to help women become successful breastfeeders and ensure developing babies get the best nutritional start in the world. For that reason what they attempt to offer is admirable and worthy of our respect; however, sometimes their approach is deplorable.

Extreme pressure being exerted upon an emotionally challenged, struggling young mother has her questioning any last remnant of confidence she has. I have seen women become suicidal due to the non-stop visits, phone calls and sit-ins of group members when they fear a women is about to give up and resort to bottle-feeding. They never seem to take no for an answer.

A client who was struggling with breastfeeding came to my clinic; she was in huge pain and the baby would suckle for a short spurt but would soon throw its head back in frustrated rage. The mother had no idea what to do. She felt exhausted as the baby was not drinking enough so therefore not sleeping and her whole body felt sick. The baby was also not drinking much from a bottle, choosing screaming all day and night over sleep. Breastfeeding groups advised and pressured her to persevere. One look at the woman revealed her desperate need for a break. She was dark under the eyes and skin pallor gave away her internal sickness. A feel of her breast revealed intense heat, signifying mastitis. She was referred to a doctor immediately. Tests revealed she had a golden staphylococcus infection in the breasts and it was tainting the milk the baby was being forced to drink.

Her other comments about how the baby was feeding brought attention to how tight the mother was screwing the lid on the baby bottle. As suspected, tension of the bottle lid caused a vacuum, making the baby struggle with sucking. I adjusted the lid, showed the mother how to check for bubbles that prevent the vacuum occurring and then proceeded to feed her baby the whole bottle. The poor little baby was starving. She immediately fell asleep and continued to sleep for twelve hours from sheer exhaustion. I learnt the lid trick from my mother when I had the same bottle-feeding problem.

In this case the breastfeeding mothers, through their own agenda, nearly stopped the woman from getting the correct care she and her baby desperately needed. Young mothers are vulnerable to the acceptance of other people in their groups and this can leave them open to subtle forms of abuse, preventing them from speaking up against the pressure.

Super Mom and Meltdown Moments

Many women enter pregnancy and the birth of their first baby with the idea they will be a super mother, able to juggle work, home and baby duties. Not only will they do this, but they will do it really well. That's the dream anyway; rarely does the fantasy match the reality. The meltdown moments I have seen from so many women trying to 'do it all' is evidence of a tough and upward battle. The sheer mind-numbing exhaustion experienced with a young baby and growing child can reduce women into a rubble of gnashing, thrashing tears, yelling and complete emotional disconnect. Functioning with peak performance is immediately challenged.

Women from all walks of life need to take some pressure off. The truth is all women, in some areas of their lives after having children, go through huge personal adjustments and challenging times, regardless of turning up at your mother's group with perfect makeup, fabulous trendy clothes, svelte body shape or the baby dressed in designer clothes looking clean and rested. Beneath the surface is a woman exhausted, rushing to remain on time after cleaning a sudden projectile vomit or bowel movement and feeling emotionally confused as to why they are suffering a lack of sex drive or deeply concerned over other aspects of their relationship.

Do not feel judged by these ladies; they are struggling like you and also looking at your seemingly perfect life, fearing that you have it all sorted out when they are feeling emotionally derailed. Honesty with each other is the greatest healer. The sisterhood of women should be making life easier for each other, not harder.

Sleep When Baby Sleeps

"I am so tired but I still have the ironing to do."

Stop trying to keep a picture perfect home when first bringing your baby home. It's insanity! Your whole body has been through an epic ordeal and needs rest. Breast feeding depletes and internal body parts are trying to bounce back. Lack of sleep is fighting against every step. Get used to sleeping whenever the baby sleeps and place a sign on the door apologizing for not receiving visitors. Become organized if you possibly can so friends and family members are forewarned of sleep and rest times.

Worrying about judgment has to go on hold. There will be

plenty of time to catch up on housework. Well, not really, but that is something that other people can help you with as you settle into life as a parent.

Put other people to use.

The best way to arrange helpful relative and friend arrivals is to put them to work. When they come over they might have a planned cuddle in mind, happy to watch your frantic endeavors to complete chores so you appear organized. Instead, hand them the vacuum cleaner and thank them profusely for the support that would offer.

Pre-warn family members of your decision to happily accept offers to wash and clean so you and your partner are free to bond in a wholesome way. In fact, this is the greatest help a mother or mother-in-law can offer. It's useful, sensible and always appreciated, unless of course you have a relative with obsessive compulsive disorder tendencies or you are this way yourself. That could end in a disastrous scenario.

Friends can help enormously if they cook a meal. Enormous pressure to juggle all the new needs and expectations that come with parenting can become mind consuming in those early days. Any cooking help is celebrated. Homemade frozen dinners are fantastic. A Christian friend of mind had the whole church create a roster to take turns to support her. They did this for all young mothers in the congregation and I was inspired by hearing about their support and obvious demonstration of faith and community in action. Perhaps your own friendship groups can do the same. However, some caution is advised in relation to ingredients that cause wind to the developing digestive system of the baby through your breastmilk. So give a list of ingredients to your well-meaning friends to better assist their support of you.

It's up to you what you take onboard. Your life, your baby.

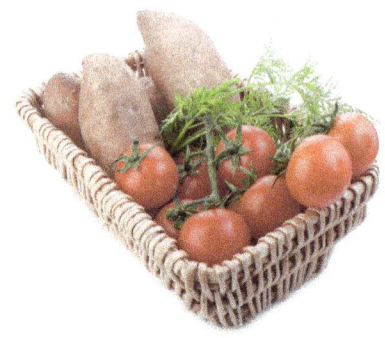

Problem Foods and a Developing Digestive System

"No matter what I do, my baby keeps screaming in pain."

For the first three months a baby's digestive system is still developing. This can pose a problem as some foods you eat might end up tainting the breastmilk and consequently upsetting their gut, causing gripping wind pain. Crying and screaming usually follows.

Everyone has their version or wives' tales about this. Listed here are the most common offenders.

Suggested foods to avoid

Foods in the cabbage family: ***cabbage, broccoli, Brussel sprouts, cauliflower***. Then there are vegetables that have an outer husk: ***peas, corn and lentils. Onion and capsicum*** can be obvious aggravates and many people report ***chocolate and coffee*** as an offender. Decaffeinated coffee for some people also causes wind; try dandelion tea instead. This does not leave a lot to eat and will require a vigilant awareness of the food that finds its way into your mouth. I know it seems rather alarmist but I can assure you this advice had saved many families a lot of stress with their babies.

It seems strange that hospitals provide all these foods, yet the baby sleeps peacefully with no obvious pain and barely even screams. Your baby is so exhausted after birth that it really does not react too much, until *you go home.*By about day four or five your baby wakes up from some magical slumber and the screaming begins. The baby becomes aware that it has body sensations and reacts to them all. Colostrum differs in makeup to your new milk and could be a reason for why your baby suddenly reacts.

I listened to my mother's advice on food with my first child until the end of the second month. I was bored and desperate for new food sensations and decided to allow onion in my diet. The next day my baby was fine with no evidence of discomfort. I was thrilled and decided my mother did not know what she was talking about. So of course I had some more that day. I lived to regret my smugness and all-knowing attitude. My baby did not stop screaming for three whole days. I was insane with stress, sobbing and begging for him to stop crying. I tried every natural remedy and drugstore suggestions to no avail. I had to wait for the last effects to pass out of my breastmilk before equilibrium returned to the home and my son's painful gut was no more. I never ignored the wisdom of my elder again.

Nervous System Maturing

Your baby may be born looking perfect and ready to face the world, but their nervous system is still in early stages of development. A baby needs time to adjust to their new bright environment. Every sight, sound, smell and body touch sets off a wild array of electrical charges throughout their body and brain. Thousands of nerve endings report to the brain by the minute and cause an overload, resulting in the need for maximum sleep.

Imagine coming from a world where sounds are muffled. Every movement of the body results in a liquid wave-like action, gently bumping into the surface of the skin, and light sensations are muted. Next minute your world turns against you by squeezing your body tightly through a restricted canal, near on crushing your head and then you are forcefully ejected into a world of brilliant light and clanging sounds. This is shocking to your baby and it needs rest and quiet time to adjust and heal.

In those early months, especially the first few days, your baby needs the least amount of stimulus you can possibly provide to help their adjustment. Being washed and clothed regularly or passed around from relative to relative becomes exhausting work. Some people will seem to fracture your child's senses more than others. For this reason it makes sense to limit access to your baby and keep the environment quiet and serene.

Women of earlier generations understood this. They would not take their newborn out in public for six weeks. Colors of the nursery and clothing were muted, choosing pastels over those of a bright vibrant hue, and visitors were kept to a minimum. These days we no longer understand this reasoning and it may seem old fashioned. Yet when your baby is exhausted they fret and cannot settle themselves as their nervous system is agitated by too much activity and stimulation.

Pregnancy and Birth: The Conspiracy of Silence

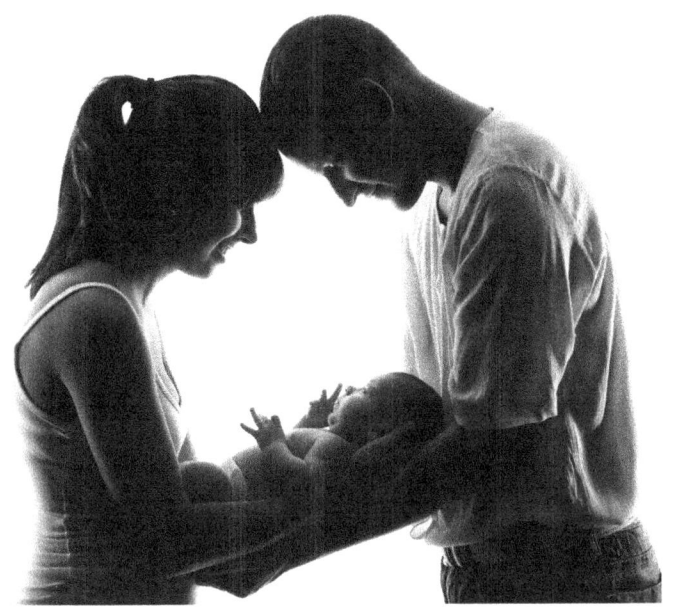

Home Alone with Your Baby

"Yikes! Now what do we do?"

There comes a time when every parent finds themselves at home alone with their baby. For a couple or single parent, the first time is when you're released from hospital and you step foot into the home. An eerie silence fills the air as you settle into a normal environment with your new baby. The realization that you have sole responsibility for the survival and nurture of this fragile child, who depends on you for everything, fills the silence. Hospital staff are no longer around to defer to or ask questions. There is no one to take your child away while you sleep or rest. This is it! No turning back! You are now proud parents expected to stand on your own and succeed with minimal training. Left to make it up as you go along.

An overwhelming feeling of inadequacy and thoughts of ill-equipped preparation fill your mind. You may even feel a quiet terror, as the task ahead presents a daunting journey of strength, resilience and on-the-fly adaptability. If you are without emotional and physical support from family, this becomes an even harder adjustment period.

Just take a step at a time. If you fumble a little, do not worry—all a baby really needs is to be loved and held a lot. Its reassurance comes from being adequately fed, hearing the sounds of your gentle voices and hearing its mother's heartbeat when you hold it close. All other jobs of running a household come secondary to this. Do not stress the little things. Just take one step at a time. If you do not have all the fancy nursery equipment it's not the end of the world. Babies in third-world countries sleep in a sling near the mother. Nothing else, just that! As long as they are loved and cared for, this has proven to be enough to successfully grow a well-balanced human being.

My Life is Turned Upside Down

'It's impossible to get my house tasks done."

"I can't even shower anymore!"

There is no doubt that having a baby fills you with delight, adding meaning to your life, but it's those other times when everything seems to go wrong or is out of control that can really challenge mental sanity.

When viewing other women taking their babies out, visiting friends or just doing the shopping, you are led to believe their life is easier than yours and she is more organized. Sometimes this is true, but without being a fly on the wall watching her every move, you will never know the stress she is under or how long it took her to finally be able to have a shower, or even if she has. Simple tasks become impossible when the baby screams, cries or moans from some form of distress. After trying everything, you'll often end up carrying them all day. This leaves no time to wash, clean, cook dinner or get to the shopping center for supplies. Makeup, special hairstyles, massages or exercise all become less frequent as you juggle sleep or the lack of it; instead, life becomes a continual zombie walk with a baby permanently hanging off your breast. Personal space is an experience of the past. All day, all night, the mind remains on alert. The job is grueling and lack of sleep is like a perverted torture. Militaries use sleep deprivation as a torture tactic. It is an effective method to turn a mind upside down and inside out until the mind finally breaks down.

From one woman to another, and as a therapist, I am telling you this is how we feel, demented with fatigue from a life turned into chaos overnight. Incredible as it sounds, remaining pregnant can become the preferred gig over new motherhood. At least when pregnant, you could still get out of the car to buy milk without dragging a baby capsule around, not have to time coffee outings around sleep and feed times, and being able to eat what you like without the punishment of three days of constant screaming. The impossibility to prepare dinner becomes a sore point, as the partner would love to come home to a perfectly functioning home and family; instead he will have to face a hostile or depressed woman. The woman feels incredible guilty that she has not been able to prepare any food all day to greet his arrival.

All these feelings of ineptness can spiral out of control, both partners feeling confused about the drastic changes a baby brings to their relationship. Men can find it really hard to imagine how stressful it is to look after a baby all day. He might gain some insight if you leave the baby with him for long durations (without his mother's help); however, he is not in your body with all the hormonal changes and the sheer exhaustion that comes with creating milk. He is not inside your brain that is thinking about all the household jobs, shopping lists, doctor visits, body shape, or coping with anxiety over a lack of libido. He might not be worrying over disgruntled family members and the politics that go with it, like you might be. He will have an earache from the baby's cry and want to get out of the house as soon as possible each day.

The one person whom you need to understand what you're going through has no hope in fully comprehending and this realization can cause deep confusion, loneliness, anger and a pervading sadness, as this is not what the media has told women. Nor have the other women we are surrounded by, because they think they are the only ones feelings like this or have felt like this—they do not wish to reveal their weakness or not appear poised and successfully happy. It's time women told the truth to each other.

Distressed Comments from Women

"I cried constantly for three weeks in shock. I kept asking myself in a desperate whisper, what have I done?" In relating that story to me she mentioned an overriding sense of doom over how drastically her life had changed as the truth of life with children seeped into her conscious mind.

"I am so exhausted I cannot think or even sleep. Every part of me feels like it is collapsing, I am constantly on edge and so angry that it scares me."

"I hate myself for the thoughts I have of hurting my baby. My ears feel pain from the crying and my head wants to explode."

"I am completely out of control. I am terrified my husband is going to take my child away from me because I cannot pull myself together."

"What is wrong with me? I am hating being a mother. All I can think about is going back to work and getting my life back."

"I love being a mother filled with so much love but most of the time all that goodness is sucked out of me."

"I am a complete bitch to my partner. No matter what he does, I have a go at him until I end up in tears and that seems to help me."

"It's so hard. I had no idea it would be like this. I feel trapped, as though my life is not my own anymore."

These types of comments are typical in therapy sessions. The best way to regain mental balance is through sleep. The nervous system needs time out, to recover and recuperate. Having a baby can feel like self-torture at times, especially when a woman's instinctual nature does not allow for her to run away from her young.

Traumatic Births with Medical Intervention

"I am so angry. I was not given a choice on medical intervention. I cannot seem to get past it."

Traumatic births can have far-reaching effects for both women and men. A woman going through extreme pain and discomfort locks that memory within her body and it takes up as cellular memory for the future. Often when severe tearing, use of forceps, followed by tugging and dragging the baby out is present as part of the birth experience, feelings of anger often arise. Sometimes it is well-placed anger at medical staff who did not listen to the woman's innate intuitive warning to take action or investigate earlier. Other times these feelings arise due to the shock and horror of how the body is affected and the birth not matching your perceived idea of the end result. This is especially relevant if there had been a completely fixed idea on non-intervention or pain relief support. When ideas and dreams do not match with the outcome, feelings of betrayal arise. The body betrayed the original ideas around the ability to birth easily, safely and naturally. Issues of incontinence or surgery to alter the damage could end up staggering the result.

Powerlessness to control the situation is a common sentiment. Men are often paralyzed by this emotion and thought processing. When they have to witness their partner go through intense pain and suffering without being able to adopt the usual male responsibility to step in and protect, it goes against every fiber of their being. Forced to stand back and watch is not in their behavioral design. This is made even worse when they witness their baby being dragged, twisted and turned in all manner of ways to free a head or bottom when presenting incorrectly or unsafely. Speaking up against the medical establishment is fraught with difficulty, leaving a bystander unable to follow through with pre-birth instructions from their partner. When they witness blood, gore, screaming and horrifying pain, they quickly defer to the experts and place all their trust in their training. In the aftermath they can be wracked with guilt and shame for weakening and not standing up. Often berating themselves, their emotions overflow in states of anger, frustration, or emotional withdrawal.

A woman processing those same events can also feel betrayed by a partner for not protecting them, resulting in a huge carry-on effect influencing the ongoing relationship. Anger can also arise toward the baby who, through the difficult birth, forced them to feel this way. This creates another potential pathway to post-natal depression and child rejection. All these emotional states are particularly evident with caesarians.

Depression Associated with Caesarians

"I feel like I am a failure as a woman."

"I have a healthy baby but feel like I am grieving the loss of something."

Throughout a woman's life she will have moved through every stage of experiencing her body as a female. In her journey she is led to believe that she is naturally a nurturer and will one day grow into a woman who gives life. Without effort she moves from one growth phase to another, the body naturally taking control of all those changes from girl to young lady, menstruating and growing breasts. Finally all these changes result in a young woman who can become pregnant, grow a baby inside her, and finally birth that baby. The ultimate betrayal and disappointment can arise when all those expectations are dashed through requiring a caesarian.

Sadly this disappointment is exacerbated by medical personnel who declare a caesarian is absolutely necessary due to the assigned doctor going on holidays around the due date. So rather than allowing the woman to go through birth naturally and in her own timing, he/she instigates a whole new formula. General practice, especially in America, seems to follow the model if the woman has had one caesarian then all other births have to be treated in the same way. Decisions like this do not bode well for the women after the birth. She is left bereft and disappointed as though something is vitally missing. In fact, many do not even feel they actually gave birth so they find it really difficult to bond and nurture their baby. Externally they behave as society expects, yet inside, deep depression lurks that makes no sense at all to them, since in their arms they have a healthy baby to love; so why the sad, alone feelings?

Celia Fuller

It is my personal theory that a huge spiritual significance and rite of passage as a woman occurs with a vaginal birth. There is some type of unseen coding in the DNA that says we must birth this way to create a child that can survive naturally on its own. This idea lays hidden and unproved by traditional methods of thinking as it cannot be measured and examined, yet women speak it anyway by expressing feelings like "I am a failed woman". "I am not good enough in comparison to other women." "I am not a real woman." I am not saying one method is better than the other, because sometimes a caesarian just cannot be avoided, as death could be the alternative. However, as a society we need to formulate a process that allows women to move into a state of female completion. Women who have suffered the terrible anguish of still-birth and miscarriage share these same sentiments and often feel a lesser human being, fearing potential judgment by their female counterparts or their partner. Self-esteem suffers as feelings of being useless and a waste of space arise.

Fathers who have witnessed a pre-arranged caesarian could still feel overwhelmed by the experience of seeing the person they love carved up on the table in front of their eyes. Visions of the uterus dragged out of the abdominal cavity to cut the baby out can become the source of flashback scenarios of post-traumatic stress disorder. The horror is magnified if the caesarian has to occur as part of an emergency procedure. The man has to stand aside powerless, but watching and listening to barked out orders, frenzied activity, and then the slicing and dicing of his partner, all in rapid timing.

Unfortunately there are not many services to support couples who have been deeply affected in this way, and statistics show that depression suffered by men and women after caesarians can be quite high and these negative affects can influence the positive progression of relationships, parenting and sexuality. Over the years I have developed an extremely effective mind journey visualization technique for all women who have lost a baby or not completed a vaginal birth. It is extremely effective and brings great emotional relief to those who have followed this technique. (See 'Wholistic Counseling' at my website: www.wholistic-lifestyles.com.au)

Hypnotherapy and other healing practices may be another wonderful path of healing for both men and women suffering depression and post-traumatic stress.

Mothers' Comments

"I felt removed from my visitors. I watched them hold my baby while I sat feeling tears of grief and trauma wash through me as I revisited a sense of powerlessness over failing my baby. The guilt is terrible."

"I cried every time I had to express my milk instead of being able to successfully feed due to my pain filled post caesarian body."

"I found it really hard to face other women who had vaginal births. I felt ashamed and less of a woman compared to them."

Past Sexual Abuse Can Trigger Depression After the Birth

"Uncomfortable and confronting memories took over my mind, preventing me from fully enjoying the birth of my new son."

An unusual and unexpected byproduct of birth can be the triggering of memories deeply buried in the subconscious. Sexual abuse has so many effects and the experience, no matter how hard an individual tries to bury it, can only be shut down from the conscious awareness for a time. Eventually life triggers the memory to surface. The birth of a baby can be one of those times of memory recall.

There are many cases where a person has experienced sexual abuse in the past and their own parent had not been able to protect them or even knew it was happening. When the child grows up and has a child of their own, a terrible fear can arise or feelings of potential inadequacy may surface in relation to their ability to keep their baby safe. Clients I have supported through this had initially faced a variety of life altering reactions, culminating in huge emotional meltdowns.

As a result of the sexual abuse, the new parent may experience trust issues around anyone else supporting or giving any care to the baby. Irrational protectiveness (from other people's perspective) might consume a mother well into the child's early growth years and even extending into a young adult life. Every person becomes a target of suspicion and great hesitancy to hand over a child to some members of the family and not others could cause offence and confusion, often resulting in partners disagreeing about the care of their child. This can be a time when major rifts develop. These feelings connected to extremely painful memories and trauma are usually not open for discussion, and fear of hurting family members causes an internal emotional war. Avoidance seems the best option, yet the subconscious mind can have a different agenda.

Agoraphobia symptoms can be common among women who have birthed a female child. Decisions to stay home and not interact with society are strategies they put in place to protect the child. A man who has suffered in the same way may form a strong attachment to his partner, substituting her to fill the role of his own mother. So when a baby comes and takes his place, it can challenge how he relates to the baby or create a sense of competition with them.

Worse than those reactions are potential feelings of fear. The very fear of being a male and if it was a male who hurt them they may fear this same potentiality lays hidden in them also, especially if he has read that many victims in turn become perpetrators.

Men who have been sexually abused may encounter a sudden onset of shame and anxiety. If their perpetrator had been a male then they could create a mental assumption driven by fear over their past abuse that they might also house the same potentiality. This can drive them emotionally away from bonding. In therapy sessions these scenarios have arisen even to the point of the man leaving the family home with no explanation causing more harm to the family than if they stayed and worked through their feelings. There are pathways for essential support in relation to these matters. Wholistic Lifestyle Counseling is also extremely effective in easing the tortured mind of victims and finding safe ways to open up and finally speak about their feelings.

Conclusion on Women

There are many amazing books in the marketplace that will guide you through each stage of your development.

With parenthood comes a huge learning curve for both partners, so it would be remiss of me if I overlooked the man's view of pregnancy and the birth of their child, and how it has affected them.

{ 6 }

Don't Forget Your Man

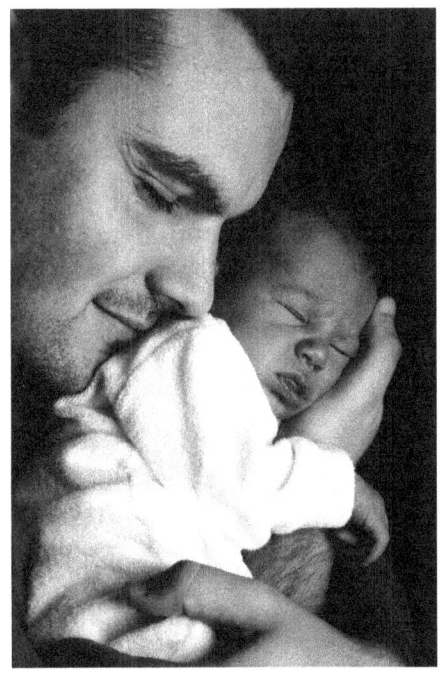

A Man's Perspective

A man may feel quite removed and left out throughout the pregnancy. He is confused and has little idea of what his partner is going through. He struggles to comprehend her sickness and may believe she is not nearly as sick as she makes out, unless he actually sees her vomiting. All other symptoms don't seem real to him.

By the time your partner has patiently waited for up to six months to see any real evidence that a live baby is inside, he has already become a little disconnected. Only you can feel the first kicks. He can only watch the awe and excitement cross your face with the first kicks occurring about 5-6 months in. His introduction to the baby via kicking has to wait a little longer. Once he's felt the first definite kick of the unborn child, he becomes quite mesmerized and this experience kick-starts the incentive to help organize the baby's room. Three months more he waits, still not understanding the sheer discomfort the woman goes through, yet delighted to feel the baby's movement. Nervously he waits, protective of mother and child.

Birth – Too Many Support People

"Why is she asking to have everyone come into the labor ward? I feel like it's turned into a bloody circus."

Men can often be overwhelmed and confused when they are told by their partner of her intentions to have multiple support people present at the birth. For a first-time dad, this is extremely challenging. Often he'll verbally agree just to keep the peace as he wants what is best for his partner. In truth though, he feels pushed aside and suddenly part of some circus act that he did not sign up for. With no idea how to protest, he often simmers away into the background. This might even cause him to become emotionally disconnected and lack excitement or interest in the whole process.

A new father has many thoughts running through his mind that he might not share with his partner. He has his own dreams and visions for welcoming his baby into the world. It does not usually feature mothers, mothers-in-law and friends all looking at the private parts of his partner as they barge past him to be the first one to catch the baby, leaving him powerless and overlooked. This is a really important time to listen and think deeply about his needs. If you want the father to bond with the child and really become an intrinsic part of day-to-day life, then let his presence in the birthing suite be a number one priority. Let him feel open, vulnerable and private in his own emotional experiences on the day. Men do this better when not under the microscope of other people who know him. This day will never be forgotten and you owe the relationship the opportunity to create this sacred connection between the three of you, or more in the case of multiple births.

Of course this may be a different scenario for single women who no longer have positive contact with the father and needs female emotional support. Partners in same sex couples could also feel cast aside, if too many people are invited in as an audience.

If you choose one additional person to attend the birth, the best choice is a woman or doula who has already had children; she will be able to ease your partner's anxiety when it arises, as medical staff are too busy to take time out and explain everything to him. Staff usually assume a partner has read the birth material in the months prior to the big day.

When a man is confronted with the truth behind the labor, he needs all the support he can get.

Celia Fuller

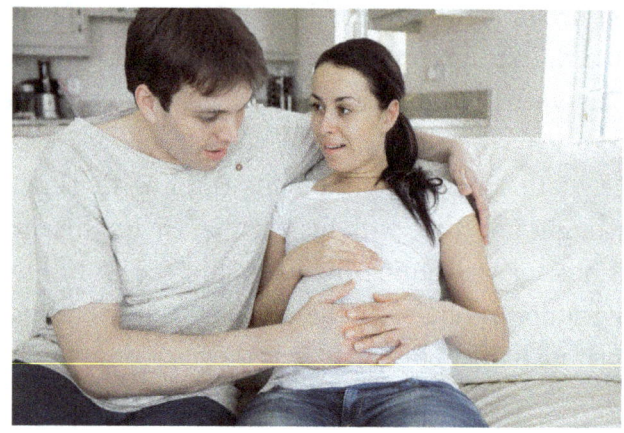

Birth Anxiety

*"I had no idea it would be so hard.
I never want to see her go through that again."*

Water, blood, gore and wailing death-like screams or groans was not his idea of having a baby. Not in his wildest dreams did he think it would be like this or that he would feel so powerless to protect his beautiful partner. When men speak openly about their experience of birth, shock is the first emotion they show. Every part of the birthing scenario goes against his instincts to protect and attack anyone seemingly doing harm to his loved ones. When a man observes hospital staff poking and prodding, eliciting a pain-filled moan, he wants to take them down. Fists can clench as he tries to remain in control. Anxiety and grief for his partner and the unborn child rattles the fabric of his being, leaving him with an impossible task of supporting easily and calmly. His own vulnerability, raw and open, leaves him feeling weak, tired and in need of emotional support and reassurance himself. This makes him feel even more guilty because he knows he should be strong for his partner, yet he wants to curl up and block his ears to the painful sound, choking back frustrated sobs. With no way to fix the problem he is stranded, alone with paralyzing emotions, wandering around the birthing suite and trying to stay out of the way.

Fathers who anxiously walk the floorboards, jump in to support their partner by holding her up, or massage her constantly, often end up tiring first. They have to accept they have weakened while she keeps going with no reprieve. When informed of medical intervention, he stumbles with decisions, not remembering the birth plan. His panic for safety overrides the rules he was given. He faces his lack of strength and clarity in relation to decisions as a failure and betrayal of her trust to keep her safe. This spell of grief and anxiety only lift with the arrival of his child, as long as there are no other complications. With traumatic births and caesarians these same issues and emotions intensify and have been known to cause post-traumatic stress disorder (PTSD) in both partners.

Baby Arrival

A man exhibiting intense delight and relief, often cries with the arrival of his long-awaited child, no longer a dream and fantasy, now a physical reality. Finally he has a chance to bond. His whole being resonates with pride and care for the fragile newborn, perfect in every way. Love and appreciation deepens the bond with his partner, the mother of his child—together they move forward to the next stage.

His life is forever changed; he's no longer only responsible for himself. Now a fragile child and mother also need his care. It's not long before he feels scared of hurting the baby with its tiny arms, legs and floppy neck, often deferring to his partner to take over, yet wishing he could feel more confident. Trust in his capacity waivers. Determined to be a hands-on dad, he continues to learn all about the care of the baby. In hospital it all seems quite lovely. The baby is sleepy and wrapped up, recovering from birth. Crying is minimal and not usually extremely loud. Nurses hovering around to reassure the mother and keep her anxiety levels down seems a perfect scenario. Visitors come from everywhere and the parents, especially the father, proudly show their baby off. This is a beautiful bonding time for all of them together. The man is not working (if he is lucky), taking some maternity days off. The woman is sleeping and resting—or so it seems to him—as he is not in the hospital throughout the night. Her internal body is trying to repair but this can often feel quite slow. Before you know it, up to four days have passed and it's time to take the baby home and settle into a family routine.

Home Arrival

"Now what do we do? How am I supposed to act?"

As mentioned before, a deafening silence descends over the home when the mother and father are left alone in their home with the sole responsibility for this new baby, entrusted to their care. A sudden realization and heavy sense of burden can overwhelm, especially when there is no instruction manual attached. They know barely enough to effectively breastfeed, there is no sign of midwives or maternity staff, the mother's body is exhausted and still repairing, and the father is preparing to return to work. An overriding sense of insecurity and inadequacy runs rampant in both partners' minds.

A man quickly adjusts by deferring immediately to his female partner, believing that her instincts will take over and all will be fine. This can be a gross misconception, as the woman also has to learn on the fly. It is true that a woman seems to quickly gather the necessary skills, lending to the idea that instinct has taken over; however, there can be feelings of emotional abandonment if the man passes over too much responsibility to her, especially when she is physically exhausted and struggling to think straight.

This is really a tough time involving a major life adjustment. Mentally and emotionally both partners have to grow up and mature as quickly as possible to handle the extra pressures that come with having a baby. It's crucial that instead of running away, open communication is imperative. Mothering is hard enough without the man disengaging, emotionally withdrawing or removing himself from difficult situations. If he runs and becomes less helpful, resentment gathers like a storm and it does not bode well for him in the future.

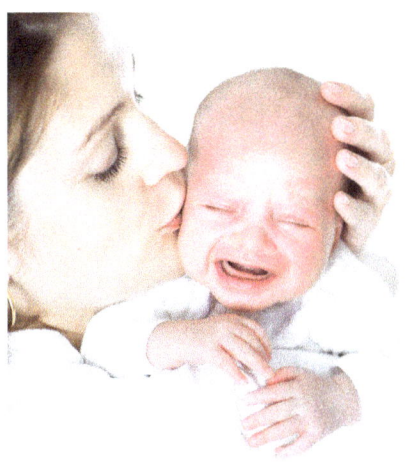

Crying Begins and the Man Withdraws

"When does this noise stop!?"

In a cruel twist of fate the baby's lungs find a new level of volume as the days of birth recovery progresses. With shock the household is turned upside-down by the wailing sounds of the baby. The mother, tired from breastfeeding, diligently tries to settle the baby. The father does his best but realizes he is powerless, as the mother, with her breasts of milk, seems to be the only way to stop the baby screaming. He watches on as mother and baby create a very special bond that he seems no part of. He feels cut off, separate and the screams are painful to his ears. Tension rises as he asks his partner to stop the baby crying and do something, anything. She is distressed, feeling her own internal shock and helplessness while she still battles a fragile, exhausted mind and not feeling like instinct is kicking in to rescue her. Heavy words and feelings between the couple begin to show. The father feels further removed because the baby shows no sign of recognizing him. There are no smiles, just sleeping, drinking, pooping and crying or screaming. The father is met with an agitated partner who has lost her affectionate sparkle towards him when he returns home from work. All he sees is a rushing, red-faced, tired person in the doorway to greet him, with a frenzied, distressed baby in her arms.

The Reality Sets In

"This is not how our life should be."

It's not long before the man realizes that this is what his new life looks like. Day in, day out pressure builds and he feels really powerless to help or do anything useful to make the family life better. This is not how television portrays the beautiful baby homecoming.

His life and outlook only improves when the baby finally smiles at him, or when sexual relations return in the bedroom. Yet even with the sweet salve of those two things, the man becomes withdrawn and disconnected from fathering. As this happens, anger, grief and resentment can often emerge within the heart of the mother. She feels emotionally abandoned, left to manage most aspects of parenting and running the household on her own. Sheer loneliness becomes her companion and with that dangerous depression lurks at her door.

The Fantasy is Crushed

The lifelong fantasy to have a child has been crushed by reality. The father is distant, the mother is exhausted, and the baby rules the roost. Friends have departed after the initial excitement, and the baby's grandmothers drift away, leaving the new mother to her business. Or they begin criticizing/helping, causing a new level of anxiety. The mother has to find a way to make sense of her new role and it does not always come naturally or easily. Many tears are spilled in the silence of the home where no one sees them. This is the beginning of motherhood and often the start of fracture lines within a once fantastic relationship.

This may seem extreme and very negative but it is important, as a woman coping with the many life changes that happen after a baby is born, to not forget that men also enter a life of change. They struggle just as much but in different ways to the woman with the introduction of a child into their life and that of their cherished relationship. The man misses the ease of life and communication prior to a baby arriving. He has to struggle with his lost freedom, yet knowing inside he has a huge responsibility upon his shoulders and thinks about this often, even if his actions don't seem to reflect his inner thoughts.

As a woman and now a mother, you have a certain skill set that men seem to lack. This is the ability to juggle multiple jobs all at once and keep track of the household and meeting everyone's needs. We expect partners to function in the same manner. Sadly it isn't in their nature to multitask or even observe all the jobs you might accomplish seamlessly. Your magical ability to handle everything takes them by surprise, causing them to stand aside in fear of being in the way. New, straight forward language needs to develop as they are not mind readers. You will have to step into the role of a gentle director, not too dictatorial, and request the help they can offer you. If you demand, yell or scream in frustration, he will only run back to the bar or shed.

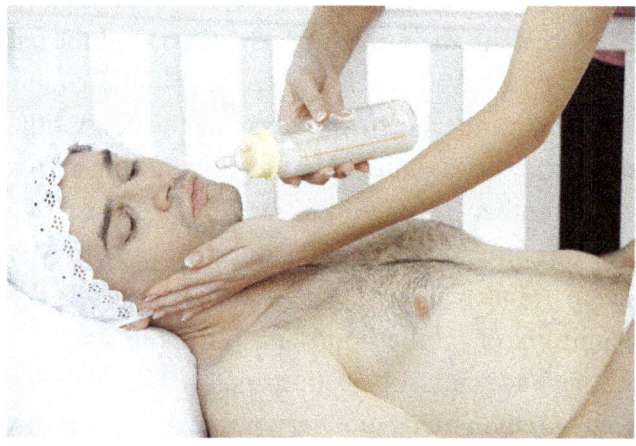

Sometimes Your Man Turns into Baby Number Two

Somewhere, somehow after having a baby, your beloved seems like he has morphed into another baby. He needs direction, reassurance and quite a bit of attention as he feels left out of the parenting equation and so seeks your love and gentleness by morphing into a child. This is not exactly true, but it certainly can feel like that to the woman who has many more demands placed upon her.

Your frustration will be at an all-time high with your new baby, so you need to try your best to be mindful of your partner's needs. When family life seems to be operating in a manageable, comfortable rhythm, make sure you take the time and effort to help him feel wanted, needed and appreciated.

I know that you are wishing he will do the same for you, but in his eyes, you are the one who withdrew from him and placed baby at priority number one. He needs special, intimate, sexy time with you to feel loved and safe as this is the way a man shows his love. When his needs are met, he blossoms and opens to hearing, feeling and responding to yours.

Your life together with a baby can become cohesive, full of opportunity for personal and relationship growth. Anger, bitterness and resentment only gets in the way of a this great adventurous journey ahead.

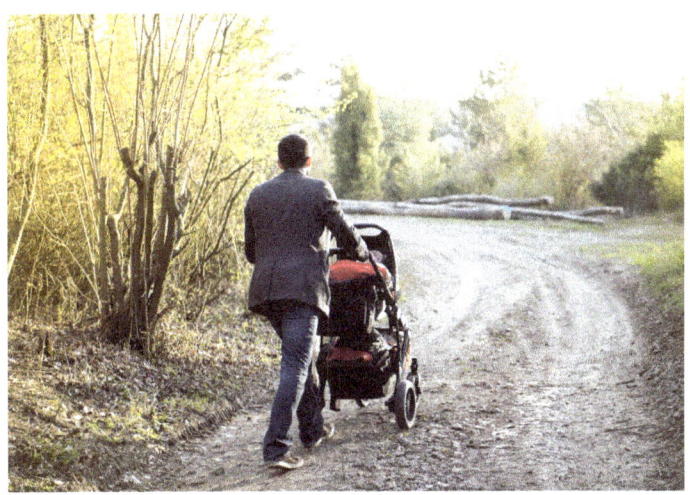

Put Him to Work

Men are practical. They love to have a job and just get on with it. He will feel frustrated that he cannot help you, so offer him ways to do this for you. Ask him to take the baby for a walk while you make dinner, finally have the shower you have been waiting for all day, catch up on sleep or sit quietly with a hot drink.

This will give him the chance to get some exercise and at the same time feel useful—and bonding can also begin. He may be nervous to be left alone with the baby. Suggest he not walk too far from the home so if the going gets tough it's faster on the return. In time he will manage and feel confident to take longer walks.

You have to be careful to not become over protective when it comes to your partner exerting a need to be involved. Those early days will cause your motherly alarm bells of instinct to go off, but you really need to show him you have confidence in his ability as a father and trust your child to his care. This will help him feel part of the team and become more engaged in his parental role.

{ 7 }

Support With Alternative Therapies

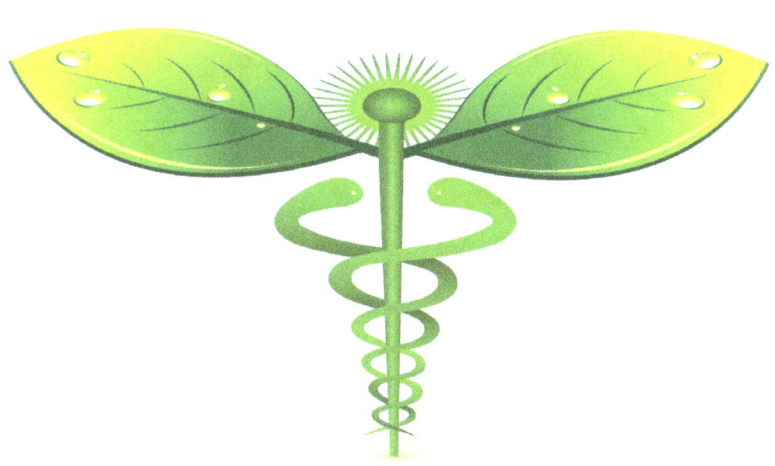

Bowen Therapy & Acupuncture

Bowen Therapy is fantastic for morning sickness, birth recovery, baby reflux, and constant screaming due to pressure in the baby's head from the birth or forceps.

Bowen Therapy is a gentle muscle manipulation technique, which acts directly with the nervous system and indirectly with the meridian system associated with the Eastern modality of acupuncture. It is a safe and gentle treatment for babies and works wonders on a recovering mother, especially where muscle strain and spinal misalignment might occur. During the pregnancy, Bowen Therapy can ease crippling morning sickness, sciatic pain or carpal tunnel syndrome. **Acupuncture** can also create pathways of wellbeing for the same issues as it works on the internal body systems, rhythms and energetic structures.

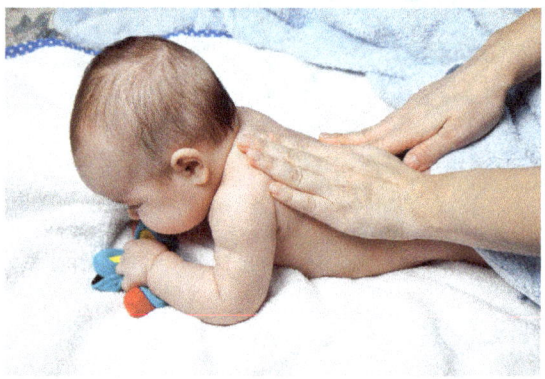

Massage / Baby Massage

Massage throughout pregnancy is a fantastic method to relieve discomfort. I have noticed that mothers who have taken time out and received massages usually have calm babies. Massage can help support lower back pain or sciatic symptoms, stiff shoulders and neck. Even pregnancy-onset carpal tunnel can be eased. After the birth this is a great way to help your body adjust and repair. Let's not discount the amazing effects that massage can bring. Deep penetrating massage can facilitate great changes in muscle action, where spasms and incorrect tensions cause the spine to distort. With guidance from a well-trained therapist who can incorporate massage and gentle stretching techniques, the body can begin regulating itself and the spine will make slow natural adjustments. There are many techniques in a therapist's toolbox to help improve health and vitality just by the use of safe human touch.

Baby Massage – Professionally trained therapists can offer massages for your baby. This can help with excess wind, unlocking their tightened muscles long held in the fetal position, constipation and diarrhea. Most baby massage therapists have been trained to teach parents the same techniques they use so you can continue using them at home.

Chiropractic / Osteopathic Treatments

Spinal misalignments after stress of birth, pelvic and pubic bone alignment, baby reflux and settling.

These therapies are all manual in nature and have their own health-giving purpose for the body. Chiropractic and osteopathic treatments release trapped or contorted spinal nerves within the spine that radiate into the extremities of the body. These contortions can occur even by minor degrees through muscle spasm or injury. The nerves that feed commands to the rest of the body through constant impulse might become impeded, causing a widespread variety of body sensations, pain and chemical hormonal regulatory imbalances.Labor has an incredible impact on body joints. Often women can end up with spinal misalignments, pelvic imbalances and strained muscles as an after effect. A baby can also end up with spinal shifts and extreme cranial pressure through the birth process, especially if a forceps delivery has been used. Possible symptoms can be unusual screaming that never seems to ease, severe reflux or breathing difficulties. Screaming might be due to your baby experiencing headaches or neck pain. Having worked for an osteopath/naturopath in my early training days, I have seen first-hand how gentle and amazingly effective these treatments can be.

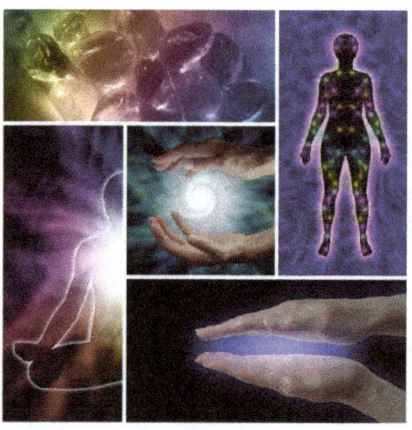

Wholistic Lifestyle Counseling and Blueprint Healing
With Celia Fuller

A powerful therapy choice for any unusual emotional problems you might experience after having a baby, this includes the debilitating post-natal depression. It's also good for stress management and anxiety for both partners.

Becoming a parent is a huge life changing event that can trigger a whole range of emotions. These emotions are often part of subconscious memories becoming triggered and subsequently rising to the conscious mind, causing behaviors and attitudes to shift and change.

As a wholistic counselor and spiritual therapist, I combine my clairvoyant abilities with traditional methods of counseling and an alternative form of healing to facilitate great change in people's lives. I do this via my clinic through retreats, and across the world via phone calls and Skype sessions. For over 20 years, I have been sharing my gift with others and the results never cease to amaze me.

Working with the person's psychology, I fast-track the sessions by using my intuitive skills to locate the core event when a traumatic experience or programmed belief system became locked within the subconscious mind. This event becomes the hidden saboteur to your success in dealing with life, love, work, career, family and your own mental and emotional processing. Through the unique blueprint healing modality I have formulated, once the origin of an issue is detected, with your permission I send threads of energy through time and space to your past, unlocking and unwinding the negative effects. This process is essentially like installing an updated version of software and rebooting your system. You are an active participant in this process. This is a powerful supportive therapy to help you not only get through immediate issues around pregnancy and birth but through all the upcoming years as you find your parenting experience challenged. www.wholistic-lifestyles.com – Celia Fuller

Naturopaths, Herbalists, Homeopaths

Great for restoring the body's balance and replenishing lost vitamins, minerals and calcium through pregnancy.

These health professionals can use a myriad of vitamins, minerals, herbs and homeopathic remedies to bring an internal physiological change in the body. Many people think they are depressed and begin to blame situations in the home, rather than suspecting underlying health conditions that could be easily remedied with simple inquiry, not needing the full force of the medical field.

Many vitamin and mineral imbalances can trigger effects within the hormonal system and brain processing capabilities. Herbs can strengthen and tone internal organs, increasing their output and increasing one's sense of vitality and wellbeing.

CAUTION: You need to be careful with using herbs when pregnant and while breastfeeding. The herbal action will enter the milk production and affect the child, and their immature systems cannot always handle them. Seek medical advice or research where you can find a family doctor who is trained not only as a medical professional but also as a natural therapist.

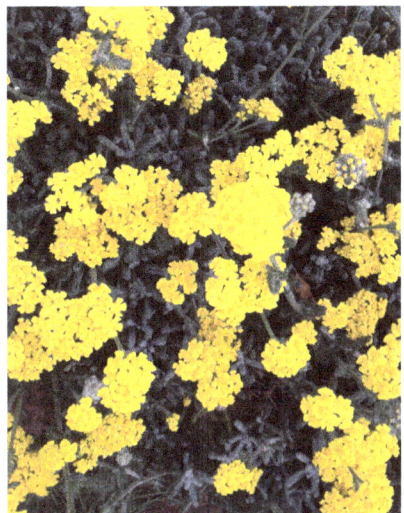

Bush Flower Essences and Australian Bush Flower Essences

As far back as the 1930s, Dr. Edward Bach believed that physical illness originated in the emotional and mental imbalances within the person. He went on to develop a series of remedies based on flower essences to address these imbalances. His remedies proved to be a huge success, and people all over the world still use them with great effect. In Australia, there is another therapy inspired by his remedy model: Australian Bush Flower Essences. These were created by a fifth-generation naturopath, Ian White.

Both therapies create great changes in the psychological makeup of a person and effect positive change in their behaviors and reactions. Some of the remedies are specific for anxiety, depression, grief and sexual issues.

In Conclusion

With pregnancy and birth a whole new reality is entered, along with a shifting world view. Sleep deprivation, crying, responsibility, intimacy, finances, joy excitement, and a deep abiding love become your constant companions. The realization that a defenseless child is reliant on you, creating a safe environment for them to survive, develop and flourish, becomes your new balancing act. Please remember, you are not alone. At least 80% of mothers struggle with the same overall issues as you. Children teach us more about ourselves than we at first realize.

About the Author

Celia Fuller has been an Australian wholistic lifestyle consultant, inspirational speaker, natural therapist, counselor, and meditation teacher for over 20 years. During this time, Celia and her husband have partnered in a natural therapies and counseling business, facilitating workshops, seminars and retreats that focus on health and wellbeing for the mind, body and spirit. Her determination to share knowledge and uplift humanity has inspired her new writing projects.

Celia, through her wholistic lifestyle consultancy sessions and sought-after speaking events, has provided incredible insight to thousands of people's lives. She has given them the tools and knowledge to assist with reclaiming their personal power and walking them ever closer to their personal success. Her unique therapy helps break the invisible barriers that stand in the way of people reaching their full potential and rising through the ladder of success.

This book is one of a series on similar subjects all celebrating the changing nature of relationships. She opens up frank dialog by creating healthy conversations on subjects normally avoided or tabooed. It is her goal to break the silence and bring her accumulated knowledge to the people who need it most and are willing to listen and embrace change.

References

www.mayoclinic.org
www.womenshealth.gov/pregnancy
www.thewomensorg.com.au
Royal Women's Hospital Victoria Australia

Cabbage leaves
http://www.lactationconsultant.info/cabbagecure.html

Hand Breast Feeding Video
http://www.nhs.uk/conditions/pregnancy-and-baby/pages/expressing-storing-breast-milk.aspx#close

Natural Child Birth
www.sarahbuckley.com

Orgasmic Birth
Books and videos by Debra Pascall Bonaro
www.orgasmicbirth.com

Books
The New Holistic Herbal, by David Hoffman
Aromatherapy, Encyclopedia of Plants and Oils and How they Help you, by Danielle Ryman
Fragrant Pharmacy, by Valerie Ann Worwood
Australian Bushflower Essences, by Ian White
Iridology - The Integrated Textbook, by Toni Miller
The Australian Family Guide to Natural Therapies, by Nancy Beckham

Also By CELIA FULLER

The Secret's Out! Men and Sex, Why Women Say No

Kind Words Uplift

Connect with Me

Visit any of these links to connect with me via Social Media:

https://www.facebook.com/pages/Celia-Fuller-Inspirational-Speaker-Spiritual-Teacher/353354161445344?fref=ts

https://au.linkedin.com/pub/celia-fuller/a1/7b/630

Your Thoughts

I love hearing from my readers so please feel free to reach me and to leave a review here on my **Amazon page:**

www.amazon.com/author/celiafuller

WEBSITES

www.celia-fuller.com.au

www.wholistic-lifestyles.com.au

In Summary

I APOLOGIZE TO ALL those in the community who I may not have represented fully with the ideas and explanations in this book. It is not my intention to cause offence to cultural or sexual persuasions of different groups. I can only hope that you may have gained some insights and converted my representations to meet your own needs.

The human psyche is multilayered and multifaceted. This book only scratches the surface of the complex nature of relationships and relating to one another. There is always room for improvement in any relationship and as we navigate our ways around each other through pregnancy, birth and the after care. Let it be done with loving kindness, compassion and understanding.

A Final Thank You…

To the inspirational people that have inspired my own journey during the last 25 years, I now add my life work to theirs.

www.ingramcontent.com/pod-product-compliance
Lightning Source LLC
Chambersburg PA
CBHW070612300426
44113CB00010B/1498